GWYNETH DOVER

A Diet for Life

GWYNETH DOVER

A Diet for Life

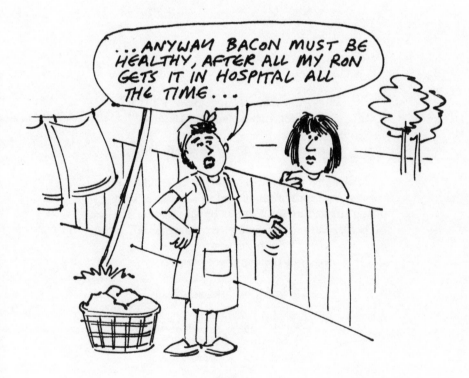

SIDGWICK & JACKSON
LONDON

I would like to dedicate this book to my husband, Richard, and to my Mum and Dad who have had to tolerate my 'ups' and 'downs' whilst writing it. Without the love, support, encouragement and bullying of Richard I would never have put pen to paper and so I thank him from the bottom of my heart.

First published in Great Britain in 1989
by Sidgwick & Jackson Limited

Designed by Michael Head

Cartoons drawn by Jon Binns
based on ideas from
Gwyneth and Richard Dover

ISBN 0–283–99856-3
Phototypeset by Input Typesetting Ltd, London
Printed in Great Britain by
Mackays of Chatham PLC

for Sidgwick & Jackson Limited
1 Tavistock Chambers, Bloomsbury Way
London WC1A 2SG

CONTENTS

INTRODUCTION: WINNING CHANGES

Richard and I were married on 31 August 1974. It was the happiest day of my life. The picture people saw was one of happiness, kindness, success and love. Yet there was another, bleak, side to this picture of which people were unaware.

Serious heart disease had plagued Richard, and all his family, for many years. Richard had a blood cholesterol level over four times the norm, his heart was enlarged, a valve leaked and he had advanced artherosclerosis which resulted in the crippling angina pains between his shoulder blades. By the time Richard was thirty-five he had already suffered three major heart attacks. He was lucky to be alive.

Our lifestyle at that time was what I would call 'normal'. We ate an 'ordinary' diet dominated by meat, processed foods and dairy products. And, although I had started to research the area of diet and health, I still placed my trust in the doctors and changed our diet only marginally. Our exercise was minimal. By 1976 Richard could hardly walk. His weight was falling rapidly. He was constantly tired. Our hopes for the future were looking increasingly bleak.

As Richard became progressively worse the answer from the medical profession was to increase the dosage of drugs. These were useless and the side effects terrible. It seemed as if the doctors were merely moving around the deckchairs on the *Titanic* instead of trying to save the ship. I did not intend to lose Richard – at least not without a fight. And, fight we did.

I began to spend more and more time in medical libraries searching out any information that was available on diet and health. I found most information in obscure medical journals from the USA as they were the pioneers of this research. We scoured every health magazine and health book with the proverbial fine tooth comb for any relevant information. Information on this topic was, to say the least, sparse at that time. I was considered an out and out 'crank' for my efforts.

As a result of my new-found knowledge I modified our lifestyle drastically. Richard stopped smoking – with a great struggle. Our diet was changed. No red meats, no processed food, no egg yolks, no salt, no high fat dairy products. We switched to white meat, fish, skimmed milk, cottage cheese, polyunsaturated margarine, fibre and lecithin. (Lecithin, which helps reduce blood cholesterol levels, occurs in many foods in small amounts, but to have enough, we add lecithin granules to our breakfast cereals.) Exercise was difficult as Richard was too ill to manage anything energetic.

7

The sad thing was that these changes seemed to be too little too late. Richard was still getting worse. By 1977 he was so ill that he spent much of the time in bed. Even the most basic movements caused him pain. He couldn't even peel and eat an orange without experiencing severe pain.

Richard's brother had similar, although less severe, heart problems and had a coronary bypass operation. It was arranged, with some difficulty, for Richard to see the same consultant. After investigations we were told that the news was good and bad. Richard was dangerously ill but operable.

We waited patiently for the operation date. The normal waiting time of three months passed without word of a date. Six months dragged by and still nothing. I rang the consultant on many occasions asking for an operation date, explaining that Richard was getting weaker by the day. After much pestering and persuasion we were given a date: 13 March 1978. We had waited eleven months. I consoled myself with the thought that Richard could not be as urgent a case as I thought, otherwise they would have operated much earlier. I could not have been further from the truth.

Richard had been placed on a 'cold' list. He was expected to die before the operation date and, even had he had the operation without a long wait, was expected to die on the operating table. He had an 80% chance of dying during the operation. The consultants could not explain how he had survived for so long. He should have been dead. One consultant called it 'a miracle'. So maybe the changes we had made in our lifestyle had had more of an effect than I thought.

Richard did survive the operation and surprised everyone by making a quick and full recovery. The doctors were amazed. This was Richard's last chance and we were going to make the most of it. Together we decided that having status, money and success was not much use if you were dead, so Richard gave up his career in the 'rat race'. My research had led us down the path of a vegetarian-type diet with no saturated fats and cholesterol. Everything was, and is, home-made to ensure that it is we, and not the manufacturers, who control what we eat.

We tried to persuade the doctors to take Richard off the 'cholesterol controlling' drugs, that were useless anyway, and to try our way – diet. After much argument they reluctantly agreed. Within four weeks Richard's cholesterol level was down to normal. The medical profession was amazed. Richard was carefully monitored for a year. He was then discharged – with a normal cholesterol level!

Today people don't believe that Richard has heart disease. He has the energy and stamina of a twenty-year-old. Looking at Richard now, even I find it incredibly difficult to imagine how very ill and near to death he was. Yet, at the same time, the memories of that period are so very vivid in my mind.

In 1982 we bought a derelict barn in the Yorkshire Dales and converted it – ourselves. The only thing we did not do was the plastering. We tried but just could not get the hang of it at all – there was more plaster on us

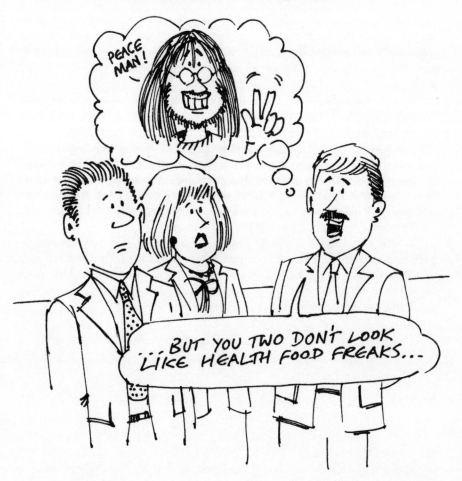

than the walls! In fact, Richard bought me a lovely present for one of our wedding anniversaries – a cement mixer. He's very romantic! The two acres of 'jungle' are being landscaped and an organic vegetable plot cultivated and looked after by Richard. He is one of the most energetic people I know. Someone once said of Richard that he was 'the greatest comeback since Lazarus' and it's true.

In 1987 Richard and I became the very first winners of the 'Here's to Health Award'. *Here's Health* magazine was searching for the healthiest couple in the UK. We entered the competition and won. That award changed my life for it made me realize that people were still crying out for information on healthy eating. I left my career as a polytechnic lecturer in financial economics and decided to write a book on healthy eating instead.

It is now 1988 and last year we opened up our home as a country house, specializing in healthy cuisine. We gently try to persuade people to eat a healthier breakfast than the 'normal' high fat 'fry up'. And the healthy vegetarian breakfasts are far more popular than the traditional with our guests. We are gaining quite a reputation for them. Some people will never change, but we have managed to open the eyes of many who have stayed with us.

Richard, I am glad to say, is as fit as a lop (flea, to those who don't know Yorkshire terms). He is not on any medication. He never has to see a doctor. He is healthy, fit and happy. The picture is no longer tainted by a bleak side. We now have a happy and healthy future to look forward to.

I decided to write this book in an effort to make people aware of the hidden dangers lurking in our 'traditional' diet. The information contained in my book is based on over sixteen years of research. I know the problems and pitfalls of changing your diet, I've lived through them all. With luck, you can learn by my mistakes and experiences.

Richard and I both sincerely hope that our story will give courage to people in similar situations and inspire others to change their diet. The pain and suffering we went through can be avoided so very easily. The major diseases are preventable, and treatable, by eating a healthier diet. Don't wait until you are in the position that Richard and I were in.

1
IS YOUR DIET KILLING YOU?

It may seem a silly question to some people, but I am quite serious when I ask the question: 'Is your diet killing you?' Most people see the western-style diet as being healthy. After all, people rarely die of starvation or suffer from malnutrition these days. And the days of widespread scurvy and rickets are gone. The majority of people enjoy more than adequate amounts of food and obtain all the necessary nutrients. Our average height and lifespan have increased – so too has our weight. The health problems associated with inadequate diet which were once rife are now relatively rare. So it would seem that all we have to do to remain healthy is carry on eating and drinking in the old way. There is no problem with the western diet. Or is there?

It is quite true that the health problems associated with poor nutrition, such as deficiency diseases, have declined rapidly in the West. As our income levels have increased the pattern of our consumption of food and drink has changed. The problem of the western diet is not under-nutrition but over-nutrition. This has led to people becoming increasingly unhealthy. Diseases such as cancer, strokes, high blood pressure and heart attacks are all too common in our society. And, what's more, we seem to accept these diseases as being inevitable. We abdicate our responsibilities, sit back and wait for these diseases to affect us and our families.

All we have to do to illustrate the point is to look at the major health problems that dominate our society today. Heart disease is the number one killer in many western countries. In fact the UK has the dubious honour of being top of the world league table for deaths caused by heart disease. Cancer, the disease that most people fear more than any other, has increased rapidly in the western world. Other diseases, including strokes, gallstones, piles, constipation, diabetes, high blood pressure, gout and other forms of arthritis, have all shown enormous increases.

These diseases are 'diseases of affluence' and have been increasingly linked to our diet. Many of our common diseases are virtually unknown in less affluent societies where the diet is low in fat, low in salt and high in fibre. Yet, when these same societies become more affluent – or westernised – their eating patterns change and the diseases of affluence begin to appear. In fact, when people from a country where the diseases of affluence are rare emigrate to a country where they are common, certain interesting changes in health patterns occur. The immigrants, too, become candidates for heart disease, cancer, strokes, high blood pressure and so on. So clearly it is not that certain populations have an inherited immunity to these diseases. The

11

major change that has taken place in the lives of these people is their diet. It is the change to a diet high in fat, sugar and salt and low in fibre that is thought to be the major cause of these 'new' health problems.

The major differences between our diet today and that of less affluent countries – not to mention our diet in the past – is striking. For one thing the meat consumed in less affluent countries is of a totally different type as it tends to be from wild or domestically reared animals, and never from those that have been intensively reared. As a result the meat's fat content is very much lower because the animals from which it comes have been far more active and have not been pumped full of hormones. The fat is also of the healthier polyunsaturated type rather than the highly unhealthy saturated fat that intensively produced meat contains.

Vegetables play a much more prominent role in the diet of less affluent societies than in the affluent West. Vegetables are used as the basis for most meals and are not thought of as being a mere accompaniment to meat. The prominence of vegetables is important because they not only provide people with valuable nutrients but also with fibre.

People in the West also obtain quite a lot of their fat from dairy products whilst in less affluent countries dairy products play a minor role in the diet.

Many research programmes have been concerned with the links between cancer and diet. In 1981 the eminent scientist Richard Doll, world renowned for his research on cancer, published a report which collated all available evidence regarding human cancer and identifiable causes. The findings were that 35% of all deaths from cancer were caused by diet. Tobacco came next, accounting for 30%. Diet was singled out as the most important causative factor in cancer formation. Yet although we hear with almost monotonous regularity about the risks of smoking, we hear little of the risks associated with diet. Don't get me wrong, I am totally against smoking and support all anti-smoking campaigns. What I find increasingly difficult to accept is the lack of awareness about the hazards of a bad diet. And, it is not that the case has not been proved. It has.

The most recent link between diet and cancer appears to be concerned with breast cancer. This is the number one killer of women and is probably feared more than any other form of cancer. Once again the culprit is thought to be saturated fat. Women who consume saturated fat, in the form of red meats and dairy products, on a regular daily basis are more at risk from breast cancer than women who are either vegetarians or vegans or who eat only white meat and fish. The link between breast cancer and saturated fat intake has been found in many studies undertaken in various countries.

Changes in our diet should reduce the risk of cancer and research has in fact shown this to be true. The common denominator in the research programmes is fat. As the consumption of fat in the form of meat and dairy products increases, so the number of deaths from cancer rises. The correlation is too strong to ignore.

The evidence pointing to diet as the main causal factor of cancer is overwhelming and beyond doubt. The level of fat consumption and death rates from cancer move in unison. And as the research continues, the links between diet and cancer become increasingly strong. The time to act upon this information has arrived.

The link between heart disease and diet is another area which has been extensively researched in an international context. Once again the results confirm that countries with high animal fat intake also have high death rates from coronary heart disease. Conversely, in countries where plant food predominates in the diet the mortality rate from heart disease is lower.

In 1947 an international research programme started which was to form the basis for continued research into diet and heart disease. The countries involved included the USA, Finland, The Netherlands, Italy, Yugoslavia, Germany and Japan. Nearly 13,000 men aged between 40 and 59 were monitored for coronary heart disease. This study found that deaths due to heart disease were strongly linked with high saturated fat intake. The result of these findings was that some countries, notably the USA and Australia, began to act on the information. The consumption of saturated fats began to fall quite dramatically with people consuming less red meat and dairy products. Other countries, including the UK, ignored the information. Consequently, in countries like Australia, the USA, Finland and Belgium there was a reduction in the number of deaths from heart disease, whilst the UK rocketed to the top of the heart disease death league. The contrasts could not be more striking.

The UK had a fairly healthy diet during, and just after, the Second World War because foods were on ration. The population had a low fat diet forced on them by circumstances. But scarcity soon disappeared and relatively cheap butter, meat, cheese, eggs and milk swamped the market. This led to a rapid increase in the number of people dying from coronary heart disease. In 1988 one Briton dies every three minutes of each day and night from heart disease and it kills three in ten of all men and two in ten of all women in Britain – hardly statistics to be proud of.

Fifteen years ago Finland had the highest rate of death from heart disease in the world. But then health education improved which led to changes in the pattern of food consumption. Less saturated fat, less salt, less sugar and more fibre were eaten. Deaths from heart disease began to fall. Finland now has one of the most rapidly falling rates of heart disease in the world. People have been made aware of the risk factors and have adapted their lifestyles to minimize those risks.

Diet, therefore, can help or hinder the chance of contracting heart disease. In 1974 cholesterol levels were checked in Japanese schoolchildren. They were found to have levels 12mg lower than their peers in Princeton, USA. Since that time there has been a major change in the eating habits of the Japanese people. Their diet has become far more westernized as they consume increasing quantities of chips, beefburgers, meat and dairy produce. In 1984 Japanese school children were tested for cholesterol levels and this time the result was quite different. The Japanese had 10mg more cholesterol than their Princeton counterparts.

Some people convince themselves that it cannot happen to them and that such research is far removed from their lives. I know that we did at one time too. But it does happen, and what makes you think that you are immune? Disease is not limited to the old. The Vietnam War brought that point home to the American population. Most of the young soldiers who were killed were found to have advanced artery blockage caused by cholesterol deposits, a situation which leads directly to heart attack. The soldiers were only eighteen and nineteen years of age. In the UK, many primary schoolchildren have been found to show early signs of heart disease. The problems are there and need to be dealt with as a matter of urgency.

We should not see these diseases as unavoidable and inevitable because they are not. Some societies have never experienced high blood pressure and yet we associate this very common complaint with old age in our society. Why? Each one of us will know of someone who has died from heart disease or cancer and yet we still go on accepting it as the natural order of things. I am of the very strong opinion that we can do something positive to avoid these life-threatening diseases. And it is up to you to do it because nobody else will take responsibility for your life.

Every single person, whether adult or child, male or female, is potentially at risk from their diet. Quite literally, your diet could be killing you and your family.

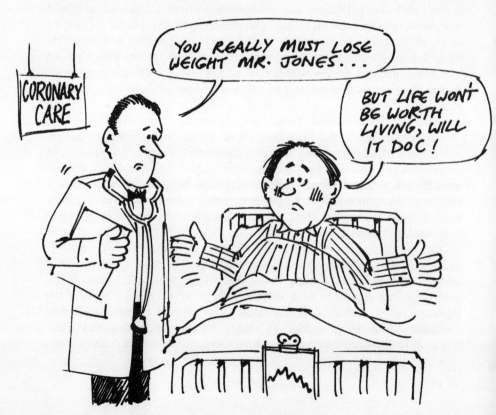

2
WHAT IS A HEALTHY DIET ANYWAY?

We have been told by various bodies, ranging from the government to the medical profession, to eat a healthier diet. This is easier said than done. Before we can make any changes in our eating patterns we need to know something about the foods we eat. Basically, we need to reduce the amount of fat, sugar and salt in our diets and increase our fibre consumption. We also need to make sure that we obtain all the necessary nutrients such as vitamins and minerals. That's what this chapter is all about.

Fat Facts
There seems to be an awful lot of confusion about fats, which is not in the least surprising. Words like 'polyunsaturated, 'unhydrogenated', 'essential fatty acids' (EFAs), 'mono-unsaturated', are bandied about glibly but seldom adequately explained. Some famous name margarines boast that they are 'high in polyunsaturates' but never tell us why this should be good for our health. We merely see healthy looking, attractive people in the advertisements and the link between health and their product is forged.

I very firmly believe that we have to understand why certain foods are good, or bad, for us in order to make the necessary changes to our diet. Most of the time we are merely told that something is either good or bad and that's it. We are not given enough information to make informed choices about the foods we consume – and this is especially true about fats.

Contrary to popular opinion not all fats are bad for our health. Indeed, some fats are essential to us. But what types of fat you consume and in what quantities makes all the difference as to whether it is beneficial or harmful.

Fat gives the highest energy of all nutrients. The term 'fat' not only describes butters, margarines, oils and the visible fat on meat, but also the invisible fats that most foods contain. Try lighting a peanut or a walnut – they burn like candles. The reason is that they contain over 50% fat. The avocado pear is over 80% fat, and so is the coconut. We can expect lean roast beef to contain 11% of its weight in invisible fat. It really is astonishing how much fat our foods contain. However, there are some foods that are fat free and these include fruits, most vegetables, egg white, sugar and most beverages. So it is not all gloom and doom.

In the UK our average intake of fats amounts to 45% of our total calorie intake. This is too high for a healthy diet. Various dietary guidelines, including reports from the World Health Organisation (WHO) and the National Advisory Committee on Nutritional Education (NACNE), recommend that no more than 30% of our calories should be obtained from fat. But even more important is the type of fat we consume. No more than 10% should be in the form of saturated fat. The remaining 20% should be split equally between polyunsaturated and mono-unsaturated fats accounting, therefore, for 10% each. Put like this, it all sounds extremely complicated, but it needn't be if you eat the right types of food.

Saturated fats are a storage type of fat and provide us with a long-term supply of energy. The energy we get from food is expressed in terms of calories and most of us eat more than enough calories to give us sufficient energy. Should you deplete your store of fat, your body will convert protein and carbohydrates from the food you eat into saturated fat. Therefore, the consumption of saturated fats is unnecessary because our bodies can manufacture their own from other nutrients if required. Saturated fats also provide us with our 'padding' and most people feel that they have too much of this already. Saturated fats remain solid at room temperature and keep well.

There is nothing wrong in eating some saturated fat but this should not exceed 10% of your total calorie intake. By eating more you are storing up ill health for your future and risk premature death. This is no idle threat – it is fact. Saturated fat increases the level of cholesterol in the blood by encouraging the liver to make more. The cholesterol is released into the bloodstream and then forms fatty deposits on the artery walls – blocking them up and restricting blood flow. Saturated fat also makes the blood much thicker, so making it increasingly prone to clotting. Heart disease, strokes, high blood pressure, various forms of cancer, including breast and stomach, gallstones, diabetes and acne are just some of the diseases which are attributed to high intakes of saturated fat.

Polyunsaturated fats are a structural type of fat and have many crucial functions in our bodies. They are essential if the brain and nerves are to develop and grow properly. They are incorporated into every single cell in our bodies. And, by making blood less sticky and less likely to clot, they keep the artery walls clear allowing blood to flow freely. These structural fats cannot be manufactured by the body and so must form part of our diet. This is not as easy as it sounds because the 'traditional' western diet not only contains far too much fat but it is also mostly the wrong type.

Because the body cannot imitate these crucial polyunsaturated fats they are called 'essential fatty acids' and we require 10 grams of them each day. Unlike saturated fats, they remain liquid at room temperature and are found in abundance throughout the vegetarian world. Particularly good sources are seed oils and fish. An interesting fact has emerged recently about oily fish and Eskimos. Eskimos are protected from heart disease, strokes and cancer by their high intake of EFAs from the oily fish, mackerel and sardines and the seals that predominate in their diet. This is in spite of the fact that their diet is also high in saturated fat and cholesterol.

Essential fatty acids have been used extensively in the management of certain diseases. High blood cholesterol levels, for example, have been successfully treated with EFAs. What happens is that the polyunsaturated fats usually increase the 'good' type (high density lipoprotein) and reduce the 'bad' type (low density lipoprotein) of cholesterol in the blood. Other conditions that have responded well to EFA treatment are eczema, pre-menstrual tension (PMT) and cardiovascular disease.

As the human body cannot manufacture EFAs deficiency symptoms can arise if our diet is not supplying adequate amounts. These symptoms can range from a dry skin to a failure to reproduce, and include increased water loss, metabolic disorders, weight loss and growth problems.

Did you know that if you use polyunsaturated fats in frying, some of the polyunsaturated fats become saturated when hot. In fact the polyunsaturates will decline by between 10% and 20% over a short frying period. If you must fry then use a mono-unsaturated oil as these remain stable when heated. Any oil that is overheated and 'smokes' must never be reused and any oil that starts to foam is toxic and must not be used.

Mono-unsaturated fats are yet another type of fat and are relatively new on the scene. They are usually described as 'neutral' because they seem to have no effect on our artery walls nor on blood cholesterol levels. However, recent research suggests that they may act in a way similar to polyunsaturated fats. The main sources of mono-unsaturated fats are olive oil and the fat found in poultry. I always use olive oil in a recipe that requires some frying as it remains stable during the cooking process, thus retaining its 'neutral' qualities.

Just when you thought it was safe to go out and buy a margarine with a label boasting 'high in polyunsaturates', there is another complication. Most margarines that use polyunsaturated fats would be liquid at room tempera-ture. But this is not what the consumer wants. We want to be able to spread it onto our bread and rub it into flour to make pastry. It has to be practical.

This difficulty is overcome by a manufacturing process known as 'hydro-genation'. What happens is that hydrogen is added to any unsaturated fatty acids present in the oil. This changes the melting point of the oil, giving it a harder texture at room temperature. In effect this makes it saturated and very unhealthy. So next time you buy a tub of margarine read the label carefully and if it contains 'hydrogenated vegetable oils', or 'hydrogenated unsaturated fat', on the list of ingredients don't buy it. It means that, although the fat is of vegetable origin and probably starts out being polyunsa-turated, it has become saturated. It will have, therefore, the same effect on your body as animal fats.

And what about those low fat spreads that are becoming increasingly popular? Well they are attractive because they are both lower in fat and have fewer calories than their traditional counterparts. These spreads contain only 40% fat while, by law, butter and margarine have to contain a minimum 80% fat. In terms of calories, the spreads contain around 400 whilst butter and margarine contain around 730. However, what we must remember is

17

that it is the type of fat that is important, not just the amount. So although we should make an effort to reduce the total amount of fats eaten, we should substitute saturated with polyunsaturated fats. Again read the label carefully and choose a spread which is high in polyunsaturates.

It's relatively easy and painless to both reduce the total amount of fat consumed and change the type of fat to polyunsaturated. Once you are familiar with the terminology you can avoid the high saturated fat foods and substitute them with a healthier alternative. It will become second nature once you get the hang of it.

THE FATS OF LIFE		
FOOD TYPE	HIGH FAT CONTENT	LOW FAT CONTENT
MEATS	Beef, pork, mutton, lamb, bacon, sausages, meat pies, liver pâtés, duck, goose, processed meats	Chicken (no skin), turkey, rabbit, pigeon, venison, pheasant
FISH	Fried whitebait, fried scampi, taramosalata, canned salmon, fried cod in batter, fish fingers	All poached or steamed white fish
DAIRY PRODUCTS	Butter, cream, cheddar cheese, other hard yellow cheeses, stilton, cheshire, cream cheese, parmesan, cheese spreads, full fat milks, egg yolk	Cottage cheese, low fat soft cheese, half fat hard cheeses, fromage frais, low fat spreads, low fat yogurt, skimmed milk, egg white
VEGETABLES, NUTS	Crisps, low fat crisps, frozen dried chips, avocado pears, nuts, nut butters	All potatoes cooked without fat, all vegetables, salads, peas, beans, lentils, with no added fat.

The Fibre Factor
Until fairly recently fibre, or roughage as it used to be called, was not a topic for polite conversation. In fact, fibre was rarely mentioned at all, let alone in company. Then in 1983 came the F-Plan diet which changed the whole concept of fibre. Suddenly what was a taboo subject became the topic of conversation in the most respectable places. Fibre gave endless material to top comedians all over the world. Fibre was now fashionable and not only respectable but funny as well. People began to talk about it in everyday conversations.

Despite all this new-found interest and publicity many people remain confused about fibre. 'What is fibre anyway?' 'What does it do?' 'Is it important?' 'How much do I need?' 'Where does fibre come from?' All are important questions which need answering if we are to understand the importance of fibre to our health.

The Committee on Medical Aspects of Food Policy (COMA) Report

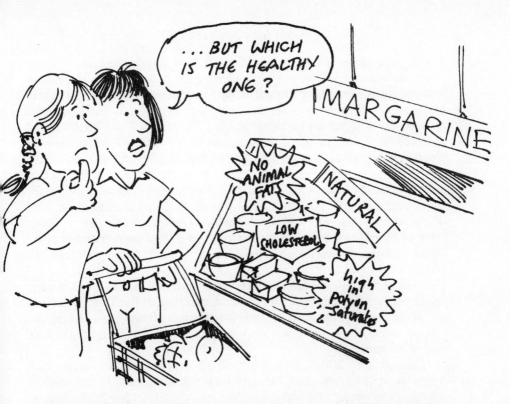

published in 1981 by the DHSS stated that 'an increase in the cereal fibre content of the diet would be beneficial'. This was reiterated in the findings of the NACNE Report, published in 1983, which stated that our ' . . . fibre intake should be increased by 33% to 30 grams per day. The increase should come from the consumption of more wholegrain cereal, fresh fruit and vegetables.' The NACNE Report stressed that these recommendations were not for people who were particularly 'at risk' but for the whole population. We are all at risk from the typical British diet.

Our consumption of fibre has been falling steadily throughout the twentieth century. We consume less cereal, especially oats and bread, than we used to and eat fewer potatoes. In fact, since the Second World War our consumption of bread and potatoes is down over 40%. Moreover our consumption of fresh vegetables, especially the dark green high fibre type, dropped by almost 20% in the period 1978 to 1983. It is no wonder that over 40% of us are constantly constipated and that over 25% need to use commercial laxatives! One Area Health Authority in the UK instituted changes to the food served in their hospitals by going over to high fibre wholefoods. The result was spectacular, although predictable. They saved thousands of pounds in suppositories.

Fibre is what is left behind once our food has been digested and is turned into faeces. Dietary fibre acts to hasten the passage of food through the intestine. And, not only does fibre increase the bulk of faeces, it also ensures they are produced more frequently.

The importance of fibre in our diet has been underestimated for many years. How many people have been brought up to believe that individuals will vary in the regularity of their bowel movements – from once a day to once a week? We have been led to believe that this is perfectly normal. We all have our own individual 'clock' tuned in to our particular needs. Sound familiar? Well, this mode of thinking has been totally discredited now as research brings to light the crucial role of fibre in a healthy diet.

There are a number of different types of fibre and each one plays a specific role in our body. The fibre we obtain from wheat and wholegrain cereals, for example, absorbs water from the gut and this helps to increase the bulk of our faeces. This type of fibre is valuable in relieving constipation. Other types of fibre, from fruits, vegetables and beans, have been found to lower blood cholesterol levels by absorbing it and aiding its journey through the body. Some types of fibre are fermented by bacteria in the gut and the by-products of this process help to keep the large bowel healthy. The quicker the faeces pass through the body, the shorter the period that toxic substances are in contact with the walls of the colon (the large bowel), so reducing the risk of cancer. It is, therefore, important to obtain our fibre from a wide variety of sources.

A lack of fibre in the diet has been linked to many major diseases with which we are all too familiar. Diseases such as heart disease, various cancers – particularly cancer of the bowel and breast – diabetes, diverticular disease, appendicitis, gall stones, obesity, tooth decay, varicose veins, haemorrhoids, hiatus hernia and constipation are thought to be preventable if fibre intake is increased. These diseases are not merely uncomfortable and a nuisance; they also kill. I am sure that every single person reading this will know of one person who is currently suffering from one of these diseases – and know of someone who has died prematurely. By eating increased amounts of fibre from a variety of foods many of these diseases could be prevented.

Dietary fibre is found in the leaves, roots, stems, seeds and fruits of plants. Nearly all vegetable foods contain some fibre. Foods made with wholewheat, containing the bran, are far richer sources of fibre than the refined milled types. If you eat wholemeal bread you are consuming 350% more fibre than someone who eats white bread. A good bowl of wholewheat breakfast cereal will give you over 16 times the fibre of its refined counter-part, such as cornflakes. Berries, such as blackberries and raspberries, contain higher levels of fibre than fleshy fruits such as apples, and dried fruits are excellent because the fibre is concentrated. Vegetables such as cabbage, peas and beans have the highest fibre levels relative to other vegetables.

So it needs only a few basic everyday changes to increase your fibre intake, without disrupting your diet too much by having to make radical changes. All you have to do is simply substitute unrefined foods for refined foods and eat plenty of fresh fruit, vegetables, beans and pulses. It is as easy as that.

Sweet Talk

There is no getting away from the fact that the western world generally, and the UK specifically, has a very sweet tooth. Sugar became a popular commodity in the UK around 1850 and consumption rose substantially until 1956. Average sugar consumption in 1855 was about 35 grams per person each day and this figure had risen to 140 grams by 1956. Since 1956, however, our sugar consumption has been falling steadily and stands at somewhere between 75 and 100 grams. This is still considered too high a level to be healthy.

According to the government's NACNE Report we should consume definitely no more than 54 grams of sugar per day. This amounts to a maximum of ten teaspoons of sugar each day. At first this maximum may appear quite generous as we tend to think of sugar consumption as the spoonfuls we drop into our tea or coffee. But the picture is far more complicated than this. Sugar is used extensively in the manufacturing of most foods – and I don't just mean the obvious sweet-tasting foods like jam and cakes. In fact about 60% of our total intake of sugar is gained from the consumption of manufactured or processed foods. So reducing your sugar intake is not just as simple as merely halving the amount of sugar you take in your tea and coffee.

For the food manufacturer, sugar, once known as 'white gold', kills many birds with one stone. It tastes nice, it increases the shelf life of food products and adds a nice texture to the foods we eat. And, what's more, it is not only sweet foods that contain added sugar. Most savoury manufactured foods contain surprisingly high sugar levels. Tomato ketchup, for example, contains over 20% sugar whilst sweet pickle has 30% and chutney 50%! That maximum of ten teaspoons of sugar a day starts to disappear rather quickly once we take into account the sugar added to foods by the manufacturers. A quick look at the table below highlights the problem well.

FOOD	AMOUNT	TEASPOONS OF SUGAR
Bran biscuit	1	3
Sparkling glucose drink	1 glass	7
Blackcurrant cordial	1 glass	6
Sugar-coated cereal	1 bowl	3½
Tinned fruit	1 small tin	5
Jelly	1 packet	19
Malted milk drink	3 tsp.	2
Packet tomato soup	¼ packet	2
Baked beans	½ medium tin	2
Chocolate toffee bar	1	9

It is hardly surprising that most westerners obtain far too many of their calories from sugar. One glass of a sparkling glucose drink and a bran biscuit and that's it – you've reached the maximum limit.

In 1983 the Royal College of Physicians, in a report called 'Obesity', stated:

'In Britain the consumption of sugar per head is higher than in most other countries and, apart from its effect on dental caries, sugar is an unnecessary source of energy in a community with such a widespread problem of obesity.'

Clearly then the message is to reduce the total amount of sugar we consume. And that means the 'invisible' sugar contained in manufactured foods as well the 'visible' sugar which we can control.

A major stumbling block in reducing our sugar consumption is that we find it very difficult to do so. Sugar is addictive and if you, like me, have been brought up on sweetened cordials and sweet sticky puddings then you have a problem. Your taste buds will find water, unsweetened beverages and plainly cooked vegetables boring and unappetizing. However, perseverance will pay off. After a week without sugar you will begin to taste the natural flavour and sweetness in vegetables like carrots and parsnips. Your palate will feel cleaner and appreciate the fresh taste of food.

Not only this, your skin will begin to look smoother and your complexion clearer. Your eyes will be brighter and you will have lost a few pounds in the process. From the beauty point of view kicking the sugar habit is the best thing you can do to enhance your natural beauty.

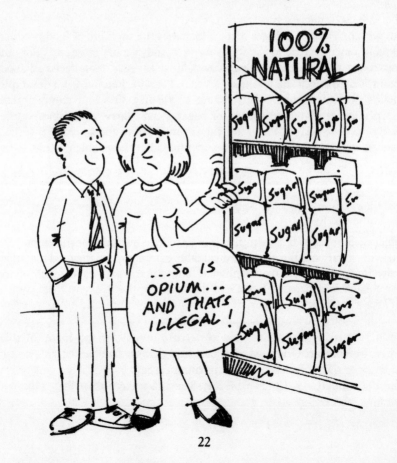

But why all this fuss and bother about sugar? What is wrong with it? The first problem with sugar is that it is devoid of nutrients. White sugar contains 99.5% sucrose and no other nutrient. Demerara retains some of the colour and flavour of raw cane sugar but is little better than white in terms of nutrients. Other brown sugars are merely white sugar with added caramel, or some such syrup, to tint it brown! Calories obtained from sugar are, therefore, 'empty calories' as they provide nothing except calories.

Sugar also encourages us to overeat and thus become fat. Our over-consumption of sugary, high calorie foods is understandable because they do not fill our stomachs effectively. The satisfying feeling of being full soon disappears with such foods and within an hour we require more. It is a vicious circle which can be difficult to break. We would be far better obtaining our calories from unrefined carbohydrate foods (such as brown rice, wholemeal bread and pasta), fruit and vegetables. In this way we would not only feel full for longer but also obtain essential nutrients.

Tooth decay is also caused by sugar, especially when it is eaten in a sticky form such as toffee. It is also thought to raise the amount of triglycerides (a form of fat) on the skin. The old wives tale about not eating sugar if you have a greasy skin and spots has a lot of truth in it.

Serious diseases such as diabetes, heart disease and cancer have been linked to high sugar intake but this remains controversial. The research continues in its quest to find the answers. But the links between sugar and ill health have been made and we need to listen to and act upon all the current advice to reduce our consumption.

Shake Out Salt

Salt is the main source of sodium in the diet. A 'normal' diet supplies about 12 grams of salt per day. The NACNE report recommends that this level is too high and should be reduced by approximately 50%. Salt consumption should, therefore, be no more than 5 grams per day.

A high sodium diet is strongly associated with high blood pressure, strokes, heart attacks and stomach cancer. In fact every population in the world that has a high salt intake also has a problem with blood pressure. Conversely, those populations with low salt intakes have no blood pressure problems. So it is in our own interests to reduce our salt consumption.

As with sugar, salt is a cheap and valuable commodity to the food manufac-turers. It is used as a flavour enhancer and a preservative, so much of the salt we eat is in processed foods and hidden from us. We have little control over this salt addition, other than voting with our purchasing power and demanding salt-free foods. Table and cooking salt only account for about a quarter of all salt eaten in the UK. The remainder is in manufactured foods.

Most breakfast cereals contain added salt – and in quite high doses. Generally speaking, crisps and snack foods have relatively high salt levels. Almost all tinned vegetables have added salt as do tinned meats and tinned fish. And the humble stock cube can have as much as 40% salt!

It has often been stated that sea salt is healthier than ordinary salt. However it is just as salty as ordinary salt and because it has larger grains you will tend to use more. So it is no better for your health.

It is better to give up salt gradually. Your taste buds will adapt to having less salt quite quickly and you will begin to appreciate the true flavours of food. If you tried to eliminate salt from your diet in one go you would probably find food so bland that you would give up the whole idea.

Vital Vitamins

Although most of know something about vitamins, it's generally rather vague. Do you really know what vitamins do? How many there are? How much you need? Where you get them all from? Whether you need a supplement? Even the so-called 'experts' argue among themselves about vitamins, so what chance do the rest of us have!

There is, however, no argument about the fact that vitamins are essential to achieving good health. Vitamins are made by bacteria, plants or animals and are needed for growth and metabolism. Our bodies manufacture insufficient amounts of them and so our diet must supplement the supply.

Although the existence of vitamins was only discovered in 1912, people have been aware of their properties for centuries. The ancient Egyptians ate foods rich in vitamin A to cure night blindness – and that was 1,500 years before the birth of Christ. During the mid eighteenth century sailors were given rations of lemon juice on their voyages to help combat the onset of scurvy. In fact, the reason why British seamen were called 'limeys' was because of the lime juice rations given in the nineteenth century. But limes have a lower vitamin C content than lemons and outbreaks of scurvy soon reappeared.

Beriberi, rickets and pellagra were also common in the past but have been almost eliminated in the West now that most of us consume adequate amounts of vitamins. Minor vitamin deficiencies can lead to general feelings of malaise whilst major vitamin deficiencies can result in serious illness.

We humans need fifteen different vitamins, all of which perform different functions and are obtained from different foods. How much of these vitamins we need is a grey area. Most advanced countries give guidelines on the amounts required daily, usually called recommended daily amounts (RDAs), but these differ from country to country. Even within countries there is argument about the 'correct' levels needed. In Britain there are only RDAs for six of the vitamins. As research progresses and we find out more about the nature and role of vitamins the RDAs are amended accordingly. A few years ago the message was 'more means better', whereas the new message is rather more cautious. Research has shown that excessive doses of some vitamins can actually be harmful and, therefore, RDAs have been reassessed to take account of this new information. However, there is a growing voice for increasing RDAs in an attempt to prevent, or protect us from, certain diseases such as cancer and heart disease. The debate continues!

RDAs are merely averages and do not reflect the fact that people will require varying amounts of nutrients. After all none of us is 'average' are we? RDAs should therefore only be considered as general guidelines and never as rigid figures. Many nutritionists argue that the UK need not bother about the quantity of vitamins consumed as our 'balanced' diet provides a more than adequate supply. However, the reality of the situation shows that we are far from attaining all the vitamins we need. In fact, research shows that much of the population is seriously short of many vitamins.

Vitamins are divided into water-soluble and fat-soluble groups. Vitamins A, D, E and K are fat soluble and stored in body fat or the liver. As the body itself stores these vitamins poisonous build-ups can develop. Excessive amounts of these vitamins should, therefore, only be taken under proper medical supervision. The water-soluble vitamins are B and C and excess amounts are normally excreted in the urine. However, vitamin B_{12} and folic acid can be stored in the liver but excess doses are not toxic. Fat-soluble vitamins are more stable in cooking and processing than water-soluble vitamins. This is because water-soluble vitamins leak out during cooking and many are destroyed by heat.

Vitamins are, therefore, fragile and need to be handled in the right way if we are to retain their value. After all, we do not want to throw vitamins literally down the drain. So, how do we solve the case of the disappearing vitamins?

Buying Tips
Ensure that vegetables are fresh when you buy them. Root vegetables should feel firm and not 'spongy' and leafy vegetables should be crisp and bright green.

Choose fresh fruit with a strong, bright colour. Fruit that seems heavy for its size is likely to be juicy and not dried out.

Buy smaller quantities of fruit and vegetables to eat on the day of purchase rather than stocking up for the week.

Use frozen fruit and vegetables if fresh are difficult to obtain, as they will contain more vitamins than fresh ones that have been stored for a long period.

Always buy fruit and vegetables when they are at their best and never when they are being sold off cheap because of age or bruising.

Buy unrefined, brown versions of pasta, rice, bread, flour and breakfast cereals.

Storage Tips
It is important to store vegetables in a cool, dark place. The fridge is ideal for small quantities.

Never store vegetables or fruit in polythene bags as they will sweat and lose vitamins.

Eat fresh fruit and vegetables as soon as possible.

Freezing your own fruit and vegetables is a good way to retain vitamins, but you must freeze them immediately after picking.

Preparation Tips
Peeling, grating, shredding and chopping expose the vegetables' surface to the air and this allows vitamins to escape. Cut them in larger chunks so less surface area is exposed. Cutting in 'thick sticks' rather than 'rounds' is a good idea for vegetables such as carrots, parsnips and courgettes.

Prepare fruit and vegetables immediately prior to use.

You will save vitamins if you wipe, rather than peel, the edible skins of fruits and vegetables.

Cut your vegetables with a sharp stainless steel knife to avoid bruising.

Higher amounts of vitamins are contained in the dark green, outer leaves of green vegetables.

Cooking Tips
Eat vegetables raw as often as possible.

The best way to cook vegetables is either to steam or microwave them.

Cook vegetables in the shortest possible time.

If you do need to boil vegetables use as little water as possible and always use the cooking liquor as part of the meal. This way you retain the vitamins that have 'leaked out' during cooking.

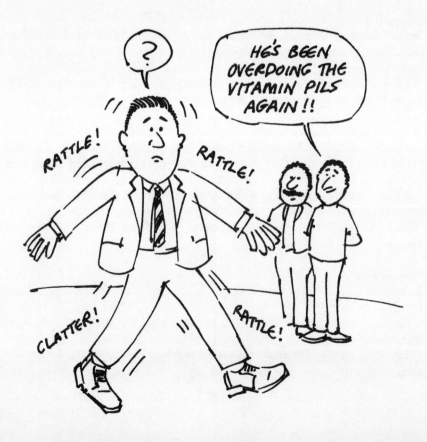

VITAMIN	AVERAGE RDA	FUNCTIONS	DEFICIENCY SYMPTOMS	BEST VEGETARIAN SOURCES	OTHER SOURCES
A	750mc	Maintenance of healthy skin and hair. Necessary for colour and light vision. Needed for growth, bones and teeth.	Depression, rickets, bone softening and blindness.	Margarine, butter, egg yolks, yellow, orange and green vegetables, peaches, tomatoes, dried apricots, cheese, milk and cream.	Liver, eels, salmon, herring and mackerel
B₁ (Thiamin)	1.0mg	Essential for growth and life. Acts in converting glucose into energy in muscles and nerves. Assists the efficient transmission of messages to the brain.	Loss of appetite. Tiredness and emotional instability. Nausea. Lack of concentration, memory loss.	Brewers yeast, yeast extract, brown rice, wheatgerm, nuts, pulses, soya flour, oats, wholemeal bread and wholegrain cereals.	Pork, liver, ham, bacon, heart, kidney, and cod's roe.
B₂	1.5mg	Needed for growth in children. Maintenance of healthy skin and eyes, maintenance and repair of body tissues and mucous membranes. Releases energy from carbohydrates, fats and proteins.	Sores on mouth corners, lips and greasy areas of skin. Skin and eye irritation. Inflamed tongue and lips. Hair loss.	Yeast extract, brewers yeast, wheatgerm, dairy products, wheat bran, some breakfast cereals, soya flour, dark green vegetables, pulses, almonds, mushrooms and prunes.	All meats – especially liver, sardines, mackerel and roes.
B₃ (Nicotinic acid, niacin)	16.5mg	Maintains healthy skin, nerves, brain, tongue, digestive system.	Dermatitis, diarrhoea and dementia. Stress, depression, insomnia and irritability. Nausea and vomiting.	Yeast extract, brewers yeast, wheat bran, nuts, soya flour, wholegrains, dairy products, wholemeal bread, dried fruit, brown rice, potatoes and pulses.	Pig's liver, chicken, meat and fatty fish.

VITAMIN	AVERAGE RDA	FUNCTIONS	DEFICIENCY SYMPTOMS	BEST VEGETARIAN SOURCES	OTHER SOURCES
B_5 (Pantothenic acid)	4.7mg	Maintains healthy nerves and controls fat metabolism. Vital link in the chain releasing energy from food.	Headache, personality changes, extreme fatigue, pins and needles, stomach cramps and walking difficulties.	Brewers yeast, yeast extract, nuts, wheatbran, wheatgerm, soya flour, eggs, wholegrains, pulses, mushrooms, vegetables and wholemeal bread.	Pig's liver, pig's kidney, poultry and meats.
B_6 (Pyridoxine)	2.0mg	Essential for growth, blood formation, healthy skin and nerves. Protection against infection.	Depression, headaches, skin disease, anaemia and pre-menstrual tension. Breast discomfort, swollen abdomen, kidney stones and artherosclerosis.	Brewers yeast, wheat bran, yeast extract, wheatgerm, oats, soya flour, bananas, nuts, brown rice, potatoes, vegetables, pulses, eggs and cheese.	Liver, kidneys, meats, and fatty fish.
B_{12} (Cobalamin)	3.0mc	Maintains nervous system, builds genetic material (DNA) and helps in the formation of red blood cells. Needed for nerve insulation.	Pernicious anaemia, nerve deterioration and confusion. Loss of co-ordination and memory. Menstrual disorders.	Eggs, cheese, milk, yogurt, yeast extract, breakfast cereals with added B_{12}, strong ale and comfrey leaves.	All animal foods.
C	30mg	Essential for growing children. Important in maintaining health of bones, teeth, gums, cartilage, capillaries, connective tissue and in the use of folic acid and iron. Controls blood cholesterol levels, maintains healthy sex organs.	Weakness, muscle and joint pain, irritability, bleeding gums, loose teeth, gingivitis and scurvy.	Brussel sprouts, citrus fruits, watercress, cabbage, all fruit and vegetables.	Liver and kidney.

28

VITAMIN	AVERAGE RDA	FUNCTIONS	DEFICIENCY SYMPTOMS	BEST VEGETARIAN SOURCES	OTHER SOURCES
D	10mc	Necessary for absorbtion of calcium from food and the hardening of bones and teeth.	Softening of the bones – rickets in children and osteomalacia in adults. Problems with joints.	Eggs, milk and margarine. Sunshine.	Fatty fish and cod liver oil.
E	10mg	Maintaining structure of cell membranes. Anti-blood clotting agent and blood vessel dilator. Maintains healthy blood vessels. Antioxident. Increases 'safe' cholesterol. Protects vitamin A. Prevents artherosclerosis.	Lack of vitality, apathy, irritability, lack of concentration, decreased sexual interest and muscle weakness.	Wheatgerm oil, soyabean oil, maize oil, safflower oil, sunflower oil and cod liver oil. Almonds and hazelnuts. Wholegrain breakfast cereals, wholemeal bread, dark green vegetables, eggs, margarine, cheese, pulses, tomatoes and pulses.	Shrimps, meat and fish.
K	N/A	Control of blood clotting.	Usually only new born babies are deficient which results in excess bleeding from the stomach and intestine.	Cauliflower, brussel sprouts, broccoli, lettuce, spinach, cabbage, tomatoes, string bean, potatoes and pulses.	Pig's liver, beef liver and meat.
Folic acid	300mc	Needed in the formation of blood cells and production of genetic material (DNA and RNA). Necessary for growth, healthy nervous and digestive systems. Transmits hereditary characteristics. Anaemia. Birth defects at conception maybe due to a deficiency, research continues.	Fatigue, breathlessness, irritability, insomnia and mental problems. Premature birth and habitual abortion. Can cause spina bifida in an unborn fetus.	Dark green vegetables, wheatgerm, brewers yeast, nuts, wholemeal bread, wholegrain cereals, brown rice, citrus fruits, eggs and pulses.	

Always keep lids on saucepans otherwise vitamins escape with the steam.

Never add bicarbonate of soda to green vegetables during cooking – it may make them greener but it also robs them of vitamins.

Never soak fruit and vegetables in water.

The buying, preparation and cooking of foods is crucial in the fight to retain vitamins. However vitamins have yet another enemy waiting in the wings to destroy them – ourselves. Smoking destroys many vitamins as does alcohol. Stress also uses up vitamins. Other vitamin destroyers include coffee, antibiotics, the contraceptive pill, aspirin and mineral oil laxatives.

Mineral Matters

Until fairly recently minerals had been completely overshadowed by vitamins (pp. 24–30). However, this situation has changed over the past few years. Research has highlighted the important functions minerals perform in our bodies and brought to life a new interest in them. But do we really understand minerals?

The first important point about minerals is that the body cannot manufacture them. If you do not obtain your supply from the foods you eat, then, quite simply, you do not get them. And it is important to get them as they are essential if we are to lead full and healthy lives. Mineral deficiency can make you feel generally under the weather and ultimately lead to serious illness. So it is crucial to know how much of a mineral you require and what you get it from.

Nutritionally speaking, minerals are split into two groups: macro-elements and trace elements, depending on how much of a particular mineral we require. If we require a mineral in quantities in excess of 100mg every day then it is classed as a macro-element. On the other hand, minerals that we require in smaller quantities, less than 100mg every day, are in the trace element group. Neither group is more important than the other – they are both essential. Basically, macro-elements are important in the transmission of nerve impulses, whilst trace elements are important in the formation of hormones and enzymes by the body.

As with vitamins, recommended daily amounts (RDAs) should be treated as a guide and not as a rigid figure to be adhered to at all costs. RDAs vary from country to country and change as new research comes to light. They are not unalterably carved in stone. And although we think of western countries as having generally good nutrition, some would say we have over-nutrition (over-eating leading to obesity), for many recent research programmes show serious mineral deficiencies in our populations. Calcium, iron and zinc are the minerals that seem most often to be deficient. These are not isolated cases but are, unfortunately, commonplace. Even people who eat a carefully 'balanced diet' have been found deficient in some minerals. And, in this country, research shows that one in four of our children are anaemic – they have iron deficiency.

Mineral deficiency is widespread. Yet, unlike vitamins, minerals are less easily damaged during cooking. Minerals are also more abundant in our foods than vitamins – the notable exception being iron. However, they can be damaged by processing techniques, food refining and sometimes by cooking.

So how much energy and protein?
After all this talk about what makes a healthier diet and how to achieve it, what do we actually *need*, in terms of calories (energy) and protein – the most important of all the nutrients that we get from our food if we are to be healthy.

The table below gives the recommended daily amount (RDA) following current medical and nutritional thinking.

RECOMMENDED DAILY AMOUNTS OF CALORIES AND PROTEIN							
CHILDREN				ADULTS			
AGE RANGE YEARS	SEX	CALORIES	PROTEIN grammes	AGE RANGE YEARS	ACTIVITY	CALORIES	PROTEIN
				MALE			
0 – 1	M	1200	30	18–34	Sedentary	2510	63
	F	1100	27		Moderately		
1 – 2	M	1400	35		Active	2900	72
	F	1300	32		Very active	3350	84
3 – 4	M	1560	39	35–64	Sedentary	2400	60
	F	1500	37		Mod. active	2750	69
5 – 6	M	1740	43		Very active	3350	84
	F	1680	42	65–74	Sedentary	2400	60
7 – 8	M	1980	49	74+	Sedentary	2150	54
	F	1900	47	FEMALE			
9 – 11	M	2280	57	18–54	Mod. active	2150	54
	F	2050	51		Very active	2500	62
12 – 14	M	2640	66		Pregnancy	2400	60
	F	2150	53		Lactation	2750	69
15 – 17	M	2880	72	55–74	Sedentary	1900	47
	F	2150	53	74+	Sedentary	1680	42

EVERYTHING YOU EVER WANTED TO KNOW ABOUT MINERALS – AND MORE!

MINERAL	RDA	FUNCTION	DEFICIENCY SYMPTOMS	BEST VEGETARIAN SOURCES	OTHER SOURCES
Iron	12mg* (F) 10mg* (M)	Vital for red blood cell formation.	Tiredness, lethargy, malaise, anaemia, breathlessness.	Brewers yeast, soya beans, soya flour, wheat bran, dried fruits, parsley, wholegrain cereals, wholemeal bread, haricot beans, green vegetables.	Liver, kidney, heart, game, mussels, cockles, winkles, sardines, herring, beef and lamb.
Calcium	500mg*	Hardens bones. Necessary for tooth formation and normal activity of nerves and muscles. Controls blood cholesterol level, aids blood clotting.	Rickets in children, osteoporosis, nervous problems, weak muscles.	Dairy products, green leafy vegetables, nuts, cereals, fruit, root vegetables, pulses.	Oily fish, canned fish.
Zinc	10mg*	Necessary for growth, sexual maturity, wound healing and sense of taste.	Growth failure, loss of sense of taste, smell and appetite, hair loss, eczema, smelly feet.	Brewers yeast, hard cheese, eggs, pulses, wholegrain cereals, rice, greenleaf vegetables, potatoes, yogurt.	Liver, shellfish, fish and meat.
Magnesium	300mg*	Essential ingredient in bone. Needed for converting calories into energy, transmitting nerve impulses and muscle movement.	Weakness, tiredness, nervousness, palpitations, low blood sugar, muscle cramps, hyperactivity in children.	Brewers yeast, dried peas, brown rice, nuts, soya beans, most vegetables, dried fruit, wholemeal products.	

EVERYTHING YOU EVER WANTED TO KNOW ABOUT MINERALS – AND MORE!

MINERAL	RDA	FUNCTION	DEFICIENCY SYMPTOMS	BEST VEGETARIAN SOURCES	OTHER SOURCES
Potassium	3000mg	Needed to keep a normal fluid balance in cells, to maintain the acid/alkali balance of blood and for functioning of nervous system.	Acute muscle weakness, paralysis, appetite loss, low blood pressure, drowsiness, vomiting.	Wholegrains, bran, wheat germ, nuts, seeds, pulses, honey, dates, prunes, milk, Brewer's yeast, dried fruits, beverages, cheese, vegetables, salads.	Fish.
Sodium	1200mg	Essential for muscle and nerve activity. Needed for water distribution through body.	Unlikely loss of appetite, weakness, mental apathy, dry mouth.	Yeast extract, cheese, tinned vegetables, most food except fruit.	Bacon, smoked fish, salami, cornflakes, processed meats, most foods.
Copper	2mg	Essential for manufacture of haemoglobin, growth in children.	Anaemia, irritability, water retention, brittle bones, loss of hair texture.	Brewers yeast, olives, nuts, pulses, wholegrain cereals, dried fruit, green vegetables.	Liver, shellfish, meat, fish, poultry.
Selenium	N/A	Maintains resistance to disease, healthy hair, skin, eyes and sight. Needed for healthy heart and liver. Protects against cancer.	Muscular disease, heart disease, cancer.	Wholegrains, cereals, dairy products, fruit, vegetables.	Organ meats, fish and shellfish, muscle meats.
Phosphorus	N/A	Needed for the building of bones and teeth. Involved in energy conversion.	Appetite loss, weakness, bone pain, joint soreness, malaise, irritability, pins and needles, speech disorders.	Yeast extract, Brewer's yeast, dried skimmed milk, wheatgerm, soya flour, hard cheese, nuts, wholegrain cereals, wholemeal bread, eggs, yogurt.	Canned fish, fresh fish, meat and poultry.

KEY: F = Female: M = Male
* UK Recommended Daily Amount

33

3
HELPING TO PREVENT DISEASE

'Prevention is better than cure' is a phrase I was brought up with. As a child I remember my mum packing me off to school with an apple, among other things, saying merrily 'an apple a day keeps the doctor away'. When the cooler autumn days began to merge into winter I was always given plenty of oranges to eat to 'ward off the colds'. My mum often tells how her mother used to prevent illness rearing its ugly head in the family by lining up all her many children in the kitchen to receive their daily dose of brimstone and treacle! Apparently this was regarded as a general health-giving potion. It certainly made an impression on Mum. All I can say is thank goodness for apples!

I have already stressed that a healthy diet will minimize the risks of contracting certain diseases such as cancer and heart disease. To a large extent we can prevent these diseases of affluence. Two important questions remain. Can we do anything else to protect ourselves from these diseases? What do we do if we already have such a disease? The answer to both these questions is a positive one. Research is increasingly finding that certain nutrients do actually have a protective influence on our bodies. Not only can vitamins and minerals prevent disease, they can also effectively treat disease. A healthy diet is crucial, however, in this process. You really cannot eat a plateful of chips and hamburgers, pop in a vitamin/mineral pill and think you are protecting yourself from disease. You are not. A good healthy diet is the base on which to build. But don't wait until it is too late, prevention is far, far, better than a cure.

Remember that excessive doses of vitamins and minerals can prove harmful and you should not take very high doses without medical supervision. Research has shown that certain vitamins and minerals are useful for preventing or treating certain diseases. However, I must stress that conventional treatment should not be abandoned but used in conjunction with these alternatives.

Heart Disease Prevention
The heart is merely a pump – albeit a very efficient one. It is really a hollow muscle that beats around 100,000 times each day and night. There are many forms of heart disease. The big killer is coronary heart disease, caused by the arteries in the heart becoming blocked by cholesterol and fatty deposits. The medical term for this is 'atherosclerosis', literally hardening of the arteries. This means that the blood carrying nutrients and oxygen to the

34

heart muscle is obstructed. If the blood cannot find another effective route to the muscle then part of the heart muscle dies. This is a heart attack, coronary or myocardial infarction – all these terms mean the same thing. If large areas of the heart are affected then the heart will stop completely.

The simple changes to your diet that I have suggested: reducing saturated fat, sugar and salt and increasing fibre, will minimize the risk of a heart attack. However, certain vitamins and minerals have been found to be particularly beneficial in both the prevention and treatment of heart disease. The protective vitamins are vitamin C and vitamin E, and the minerals are calcium, magnesium and potassium. Diets rich in these nutrients will offer some protection against heart disease.

Cholesterol

A few years ago the medical profession was divided as to the importance of cholesterol in causing blocked arteries. Today there can be no doubt about it. Raised cholesterol levels are a major cause of heart disease. Cholesterol is a fatty substance that clings to the artery walls, thereby narrowing them. This not only restricts the blood flow but also makes the blood more prone to clotting. There are two main types of cholesterol, one of which is 'good' and one 'bad'. Low density lipoprotein, or LDL for short, is the trouble-maker. This is the one that blocks the arteries and causes the problems. The 'good' type, 'high density lipoprotein', or HDL, actually reduces the bad type in the blood. So what we want is a high level of HDL and a low level of LDL as this will protect against heart disease.

Increasing the consumption of polyunsaturated fatty acids will tend to increase the level of HDL. Vitamin E has been shown to protect polyunsaturated fatty acids in the blood from being destroyed, so increasing the level of the 'good' HDL type of cholesterol. Raised blood cholesterol levels have been reduced by taking vitamin C or nicotinic acid (niacin) daily.

Strokes

A stroke is usually caused by atherosclerosis of brain arteries or high blood pressure. The brain is damaged and usually this results in paralysis down one side of the body. Once again a switch from saturated to polyunsaturated fatty acids is desirable. The vitamins C and E have also been shown to be useful both as a preventative measure and in treatment of the condition.

High Blood Pressure

Blood pressure is the force generated by the blood within the system of arteries. When blood pressure is measured it is expressed by two figures. The first figure shows the 'systolic' pressure, the pressure of the blood leaving the heart. The second figure is the 'diastolic' pressure, the pressure in the artery itself. Blood pressure readings are expressed as the systolic over the diastolic. A normal reading would be about 120/80.

Many factors, such as narrowing of the arteries, weight gain and kidney problems, can cause the pressure of blood to rise. This is a problem because it can result in a heart attack or a stroke. In addition to a healthy diet a high ratio of potassium to sodium has been found very effective in reducing high blood pressure. A diet rich in potassium and low in sodium is, therefore, particularly useful in preventing or treating high blood pressure. Research studies have also shown that increasing the consumption of foods rich in the minerals calcium and magnesium can be beneficial.

Cancer Prevention

Cancer arises when cells divide in an abnormal and uncontrollable manner, which leads to the development of malignant cells. Cancer cells travel around the body in the bloodstream and this spreads the cancer to other parts of the body. Tumours that do not spread are called benign. Recent research indicates that cancer is made up of two stages. The first stage is 'initiation' and the second stage is 'promotion'. Carcinogenic (cancer forming) factors which are widespread in the environment, such as radiation and exhaust fumes, change the genetic blueprint of cells in the first stage. The second stage is then necessary if malignancy is to develop. Diet, especially high saturated fat intake, is considered to be the most important factor in this second stage of cancer.

In scientific trials vitamins A, C and E have been found to act as protectors against cancer. Vitamin A actually suppresses the formation of malignant cells whilst vitamins C and E act to block the formation of carcinogens from food. Calcium has been found to be of some use in the prevention of cancer of the colon. It acts like a sponge to absorb excess bile acids, caused by high fat intake, and thus protects the wall of the bowel. More recently, a trace mineral called selenium has been found to be of particular use in preventing *and* treating cancer. It appears that selenium acts in two ways. It boosts our own immune system, giving us extra protection from cancer, and also toughens the membranes of the cells making them less prone to attack.

Reducing the risk of these life-threatening diseases is possible by simply being aware of the 'good' and 'bad' foods in your diet and taking the appropriate action.

4
THE PROOF OF THE PUDDING

All the recipes contained in this book have one very important thing in common – they are good for your health. Each recipe is healthy in its own right in terms of providing nutrients, being low in fat, salt and sugar and high in fibre. They do, therefore, fall in line with current thinking on healthy diets. By the way, when I use the word 'diet' I mean it in the broadest sense – the food we consume. As soon as you mention the word 'diet' most people assume that you are talking about slimming. I am not. However, you will find that with a healthy wholefood diet you will tend not to put on weight. In fact, if anything, you will lose any surplus weight you may have.

The recipes range from tempting starters to delicious desserts. There is something for everyone to try and enjoy. And, although each recipe is vegetarian or vegan, I am not waving the vegetarian banner in order to persuade everyone to become a total vegetarian. I am perfectly happy being vegetarian but people have minds of their own, and at the end of the day, they make their own choices about diet. I see this book as providing another option. People don't have to be strictly categorized as 'meat eaters' or 'vegetarians'. You can eat both vegetarian food and meat-based foods – they are not, as many people believe, mutually exclusive. The important factor is that you eat a diet which is healthier; and this means cutting down as much as possible on meat consumption. The recipes contained in this book provide you with the information and knowledge to do this effectively. And whether you choose healthy vegetarian alternatives for all your meals or just two or three a week, you will be achieving a healthier diet for yourself and your family.

If you do consume meat always make sure that you cook it with 'fat minimization' in mind. Trim the fat off any meat before you cook it. When cooking meat never let it stand in its own fat and juices – as you would in roasting and frying. Better ways to cook it would be grilling, baking on a trivet or steaming. These methods ensure that a lot of the fat content is 'cooked out' of the meat and can be thrown away. Never use this mixture of fat and juices for gravy as it is full of saturated fat and cholesterol. Remember that fish and white meats, such as chicken and turkey (but always remove the skin before cooking as this is where most of the fat is contained), are far far healthier than red meats.

The Recipes
You will be familiar with most of the ingredients used in the recipes.

However, occasionally you may come across something which you have neither seen nor used before. For example, tahini, which is sesame seed paste, silken tofu, which is a soya bean curd, and concentrated soya milk. You may not find these on the supermarket shelves, although some large stores do stock them, but they are easily obtained from good healthfood shops.

Each of the recipes contains a row of symbols to tell you, at a glance, about freezing etc. The key to this row of symbols is:

F   Suitable for freezing   4   Number of servings   V   Suitable for vegans

Nutrition boxes
A 'nutrition box' is also given for each recipe to give you some idea of the nutrients it contains. This box not only gives the calorific value of each serving but also the recommended daily amounts (RDA's) for major nutrients. The diagram below gives a detailed explanation of the 'nutrition box'.

The amount of a particular nutrient, per serving, contained in this recipe.

The figures in this column show the proportion of RDA given in the recipe, per serving.

The nutrients

Information not available.

Calories based on 2500. Protein based on 62.5g.

NUTRITION BOX (per serving)					
	Quantity	% RDA		Quantity	% RDA
Calories	576	23.1	Copper	1.1mcg	57.4
Protein	33.8g	54.0	Zinc*	3.7mcg	36.8
Total Fat	24.1g	32.2	Vitamin A*	1690.5mg	225.4
made up of:			Vitamin C*	42.0mg	140.0
Saturated	4.1g		Vitamin D	1.5mcg	15.3
Polyunsat.	10.8g	–	Vitamin E	29.8mg	248.0
Mono-unsat.	3.8g	–	Vitamin B₁*	.6mg	62.9
Cholesterol	–	–	Vitamin B₂*	.4mg	30.2
Fibre	80.3g	80.3	Nicotinic Acid*	8.3mg	50.5
Iron*	16.3mg	158.2	Vitamin B₆	1.5mg	74.5
Calcium*	1026.3mg	205.3	Vitamin B₁₂	1.3mcg	64.4
Magnesium*	223.0mg	74.3	Folic Acid	263.2mg	87.7
Potassium	1975.5mg	65.8	Starch	51.7g	–
Sodium	577.0mg	48.1	Sugars	51.5g	–

USEFUL FOR:

CANCER PREVENTION, HEART DISEASE PREVENTION, STROKE PREVENTION. HYPERTENSION REDUCTION, CHOLESTEROL REDUCTION.

Research shows that certain nutrients are useful in preventing or treating certain diseases. Each nutrition box indicates those diseases that will benefit from the nutrients contained in this particular recipe.

The 'recommended daily amount', or RDA, for nutrients varies from country to country. Where the UK suggests RDAs I have used their average figure as a base. These nutrients are marked ★ in the nutrition box opposite. The remaining nutrients are based on an average of the combined suggested RDAs from other countries. RDAs should only be used as a guideline; see Chapter 2 'What is a Healthy Diet Anyway?'.

Conversion recipes
You will find that at the start of some of the following chapters I have given examples of how you can convert traditional recipes to newer, healthier versions. Obviously this isn't necessary for things like salads – though keep away from the mayonnaise and salad cream – but I hope it will help you to see the principles involved and enable you to convert favourite recipes.

Conversion tables
If you're anything like me you will still be totally confused when trying to use metric weights and measures. I still think in the old pounds and ounces. Throughout the book, however, I have given both the metric and imperial measurements for weights and measurements. All you need to remember is to keep to either one or the other and you should be all right. The following table gives you the equivalents. And, as you will no doubt notice, for some

MEASUREMENT EQUIVALENTS			
Grams (g)	Ounces (oz)	Milliletres (ml)	Fluid Ounces (fl. oz)
25	1	25	1
40	1½	50	2
50	2	75	3
60	2½	125	4
75	3	150	5 (¼ pint)
100	4	175	6
125	4	200	7
150	5	225	8
175	6	250	10 (½ pint)
200	7	275	10 (½ pint)
225	8	300	11
250	9	350	12
275	10	375	13
300	11	400	15 (¾ pint)
350	12	425	16 (¾ pint)
375	13	450	17
400	14	475	18
425	15	500	20 (1 pint)
450	16	550	20 (1 pint)
475	17	575	30
500	18	850	35
700	24	1000	40
1000	2 pounds	1.2 litres	

of the imperial weights there are two possible metric equivalents. This metrication lark is so straightforward! You will find that in my recipes I sometimes use one of the equivalents and then sometimes the other. It all depends which is better for the particular recipe.

The tablespoons and teaspoons used in my recipes are the standard sizes, 15ml and 5ml respectively, and are level, not heaped.

CENTIMETRES TO INCHES	
Centimetres	Inches
6mm	¼in
1cm	½in
2.5cm	1in
5cm	2in
7.5cm	3in
10cm	4in
12.5cm	5in
15cm	6in
18cm	7in
20cm	8in
23cm	9in
25cm	10in
28cm	11in
30cm	12in

OVEN TEMPERATURES			
Temperature	Centigrade (C)	Fahrenheit (F)	Gas Mark (GM)
	70	150	
	80	175	
	100	200	
VERY COOL	110	225	¼
	120	250	½
	140	275	1
COOL	150	300	2
WARM	160	325	3
	180	350	4
FAIRLY HOT	190	375	5
	200	400	6
	220	425	7
HOT	230	450	8
VERY HOT	240	475	9
	260	500	9

Ovens can vary enormously, and you will probably know any little quirks that yours has. It is important to remember that oven temperatures given in recipes are a guide. You know your oven better than anyone else, so if you know it is a particularly hot one it is best to set it slightly lower than the recipe suggests. And, of course, the reverse is equally true. If yours is a cool oven, up the temperature from that given in the recipe.

North American readers may be unfamiliar with some of our ingredients as we call them something different in the UK. These are all mentioned in the following recipes.

INGREDIENTS	
UK NAME	AMERICAN NAME
Aubergine	Egg plant
Courgette	Zucchine
Biscuits	Cookies
Onion	Bermuda Onion
Spring onion	Scallion
Marrow	Squash

NORTH AMERICAN MEASUREMENT EQUIVALENTS		
1 pint/575ml		2¼ cups
1oz /25g	margarine	2 tbsp
1oz /25g	flour	2 tbsp
1oz /25g	chopped seeds	2 tbsp
1oz /25g	grated cheese	4 tbsp
1lb /450g	breadcrumbs	8 cups
1lb /450g	rice (uncooked)	2 cups
1lb /450g	wholemeal flour	4 cups
1lb /450g	mashed potato	2 cups
1lb /450g	small beans	2 cups
1lb /450g	large beans	3 cups
1lb /450g	ground seeds	4 cups
1lb /450g	cottage cheese	2 cups
1lb /450g	soft cheese	2 cups

Stock

The secret of many tasty, well-flavoured dishes lies in the stock that you use. Do avoid commercial stock cubes if you can; home-made stock, as in so many other things, is best and you can avoid using salt which bought stock cubes contain.

Onions, garlic, freshly ground black pepper and enough boiling water to cover them form the basis of all my stocks. Bring to the boil and then simmer until the vegetables are soft. If you want a thin stock strain off the vegetables and throw them away, and just use the liquid in which they have been cooked. For a thicker stock, perhaps for a casserole or thick soup, put the stock, vegetables and all, through a sieve or liquidizer. Although you can add other vegetables to the basic ingredients – leeks and carrots are good – avoid cabbage which can be unpleasantly strong and potatoes which are apt to break up.

5
TEMPTING BEGINNINGS

To me the starter is the most important part of any meal. Not because I particularly enjoy the starter more than the other courses but because it sets the tone for what is to follow. Remember the old saying 'first impressions are important'? It applies to food just as much as to anything else.

Any starter should tempt and tantalize the taste buds – hence the title of this chapter. It should make you long for the next course and not be looked upon as something to get through in order to progress to the rest of the meal. I always try to make interesting starters that intrigue people. But that does not mean that you have to spend ages preparing them. Most of the starters in this chapter are very easy and quick to make and freeze very well. What I tend to do is make double quantities of our favourites and freeze them – it makes life so much easier.

Soups remain the faithful standby for the vegetarian, but the scope is much wider than this. Remember that soups, especially when home-made, tend to be quite substantial and so only small portions are necessary. I love a nice hearty soup but then often find that I am too full to enjoy the main course! Many soups, if served with garlic bread or dumplings, are main courses in themselves and are wonderful served on a cold, wintry day. However, soups should not be limited to the cold winter months when the main ingredients are root crops. Summer soups are refreshing, served hot or chilled, and make use of seasonal vegetables such as spinach and lettuce.

In this chapter you will find some interesting soup recipes and also some tasty alternatives. For instance, vegetarian pâtés which rely on ingredients such as mushrooms and seeds rather than chicken livers. To many people a vegetarian pâté is unthinkable but it isn't, as you'll see. These pâtés also make very good sandwich fillings and are useful served with salads as a main course or snack.

I cannot stress the importance of presentation often enough. Think of the plate, or dish, as a painting palette to be filled with either bursts of colour or gentle blends of colour. And don't forget that textures and shapes make the dish even more interesting both to look at and to eat.

Common problems
The only problem that I can think of associated with starters is lack of imagination. A thick vegetable soup or chilled melon boat seem 'safe' starters but are really terribly boring. Try making soups which are light, delicate and have a subtle blend of flavours. Think about serving chilled soups –

they are wonderfully refreshing on a warm summer's day. Instead of eating wholemeal bread with the soup try hot poppy seed rolls (page 125). Melon is a good starter to any meal as it cleanses the palette and gets the old taste buds ready for action. Chop the melon into chunks and combine it with other things, such as fruits, spices and cheeses, instead of the traditional boat theme. It makes a welcome change.

Conversion recipes

Most people can make vegetable soups without any problem at all and not very much 'conversion' is required. The obvious ingredient which needs changing in vegetable soup dishes is chicken stock and you simply replace this with vegetable stock. However, more subtle changes are needed in some recipes which use cream and full fat milk for 'lighter' soups. But once again the changes are simple and do not detract from the taste.

Pâtés take a little bit more effort to 'convert' but are well worth it. The meat element is easily replaced with ingredients like mushrooms and pulses and the egg yolks are simply not needed. Tofu and low fat soft cheeses are used instead of any cream listed in a recipe. The following 'conversion' recipes will show you exactly what I mean.

TRADITIONAL RECIPE	CONVERSION RECIPE
Vichyssoise	**Vichyssoise**
3 leeks	3 leeks
1 onion	1 onion
1lb/500g potatoes	1lb/500g potatoes
2oz/50g butter	2oz/50g extra virgin olive oil
1½pt/575ml chicken stock	1½pt/575ml vegetable stock
salt	low sodium salt
pepper	black pepper
½pt/250ml single cream	½pt/250ml silken tofu
Chopped Liver Pâté	**Chopped Mushroom Pâté**
2oz/50g butter	2oz/50g polyunsaturated margarine, unhydrogenated
1 onion	1 onion
6oz/175g chicken livers	6oz/175g mushrooms
1 garlic clove	1 garlic clove
salt	low sodium salt
pepper	black pepper
2 eggs	2 egg whites

Cream of barley soup (F V 4)

Richard has always loved barley in soups and hot pots, which is a good thing as it is extremely good for the heart. Pot barley is unrefined pearl barley and therefore contains more nutrients and fibre.

Preparation time 20 minutes
Cooking Time 100 minutes
Ingredients: Imperial/Metric

2 tbsp	pot barley, washed
10fl oz/275ml	vegetable stock
1	onion, peeled and chopped
½tsp	celery seeds
1	bay leaf
1oz/25g	polyunsaturated margarine (unhydrogenated)
2tbsp	wholemeal flour
20fl oz/500ml	soya milk (sugar free)
	black pepper and low sodium salt

Method

1 Simmer the barley in the stock for about 1 hour.
2 Add the onion, celery seeds and bay leaf and cook for a further 30 minutes.
3 Melt the margarine in a saucepan and add the flour. Cook for 1 minute, stirring.
4 Remove from the heat and gradually stir in the milk.
5 Add to the barley mixture.
6 Remove the bay leaf.
7 Reheat, stirring, and season. Serve with garlic bread.

NUTRITION BOX (per serving)					
	Quantity	% RDA		Quantity	% RDA
Calories	188	7.5	Copper	0.1mcg	5.8
Protein	8.8g	14.1	Zinc	0.7mcg	7.4
Total fat	8.3g	11.1	Vitamin A	56.3mg	7.5
made up of:			Vitamin C	8.2mg	27.5
saturated	1.4g	–	Vitamin D	0.5mcg	4.9
polyunsat.	5.5g	–	Vitamin E	1.7mg	14.1
mono-unsat.	1.3g	–	Vitamin B$_1$	0.3mg	34.9
Cholesterol	–	–	Vitamin B$_2$	0.3mg	20.5
Fibre	3.2g	10.6	Nicotinic acid	2.7mg	16.4
Iron	5.3mg	51.3	Vitamin B$_6$	0.7mg	43.1
Calcium	118.3mg	23.7	Vitamin B$_{12}$	0.8mcg	40.6
Magnesium	56.6mg	18.9	Folic Acid	13.4mg	4.5
Potassium	218.4mg	7.8	Starch	16.8g	–
Sodium	62.6mg	5.2	Sugars	47.6g	–
USEFUL FOR: CHOLESTEROL REDUCTION: DAIRY FOOD ALLERGY DIETS.					

Leek and butter bean soup (F V 4)

Leeks and butter beans go particularly well together and the rosemary adds a lovely aromatic quality.

Preparation time 30 minutes
Cooking time: 75 minutes
Ingredients: Imperial/Metric

1oz/25g	polyunsaturated margarine (unhydrogenated)
1	onion, peeled and chopped
2	leeks, washed carefully and sliced
4oz/125g	butter beans, soaked and drained
1tbsp	dried rosemary
1½pts/575ml	vegetable stock (unsalted)
4tbsp	concentrated soya milk (sugar free)
	black pepper and low sodium salt
	watercress to garnish

Method

1 Melt the margarine in a large saucepan and fry the onion and leeks for about 10 minutes
2 Add the beans, rosemary and stock.
3 Bring to the boil and simmer for 1 hour, until the beans are cooked.
4 Add the concentrated soya milk and liquidize until smooth.
5 Add the seasoning.
6 Reheat and serve garnished with watercress.

NUTRITION BOX (per serving)					
	Quantity	% RDA		Quantity	% RDA
Calories	94.1	3.8	Copper	0.2mcg	11.9
Protein	5.5g	8.7	Zinc	0.5mcg	4.9
Total fat	3.3g	4.4	Vitamin A	30.1mg	4.0
made up of:			Vitamin C	11.9mg	39.5
saturated	0.7g	–	Vitamin D	0.2mcg	2.5
polyunsat.	1.8g	–	Vitamin E	1.0mg	8.4
mono-unsat.	0.6g	–	Vitamin B_1	0.3mg	27.2
Cholesterol	–	–	Vitamin B_2	0.2mg	16.5
Fibre	4.6g	15.2	Nicotinic Acid	2.8mg	16.9
Iron	3.8mg	36.4	Vitamin B_6	0.3mg	16.8
Calcium	57.3mg	11.4	Vitamin B_{12}	0.6mcg	28.7
Magnesium	35.2mg	11.7	Folic Acid	17.2mg	5.7
Potassium	394.4mg	13.1	Starch	7.3g	–
Sodium	41.0mg	3.4	Sugars	3.6g	–
USEFUL FOR: HYPERTENSION REDUCTION; DAIRY FOOD ALLERGY DIETS; COELIACS.					

Lettuce soup (F V 4)

A very economical soup to make in summer when lettuces are plentiful. A delicate green in colour, the soup looks very attractive with the spring onions sprinkled on the top. Can be eaten hot or chilled.

Preparation time: 20 minutes
Cooking time: 55 minutes
Ingredients: Imperial/Metric

2oz/50g	polyunsaturated margarine (unhydrogenated)
12oz/350g	lettuce leaves, washed and chopped
4	spring onions, washed and chopped
1tbsp	wholemeal flour
20fl oz/500ml	vegetable stock
5fl oz/150ml	soya milk
	black pepper and low sodium salt

Method

1 Melt the margarine in a large saucepan and fry the lettuce and all but a teaspoon of the chopped spring onions for 5 minutes.
2 Stir in the flour and add the stock.
3 Bring to the boil and simmer for 45 minutes, covered.
4 Liquidize the soup until smooth.
5 Add the soya milk and seasoning.
6 Reheat, but do not boil.
7 Serve hot with the remaining chopped spring onions scattered on top.

NUTRITION BOX (per serving)					
	Quantity	% RDA		Quantity	% RDA
Calories	151.7	6.1	Copper	0.1mcg	3.4
Protein	4.8g	7.7	Zinc	0.4mcg	3.7
Total fat	11.8g	15.7	Vitamin A	258.6mg	34.5
made up of:			Vitamin C	26.9mg	89.6
saturated	2.6g	–	Vitamin D	1.0mcg	9.9
polyunsat.	6.1g	–	Vitamin E	3.6mg	30.2
mono-unsat.	2.5g	–	Vitamin B_1	0.4mg	42.1
Cholesterol	–	–	Vitamin B_2	0.5mg	32.0
Fibre	2.3g	7.5	Nicotinic acid	3.7mg	22.3
Iron	6.0mg	58.0	Vitamin B_6	0.3mg	16.5
Calcium	67.9mg	13.6	Vitamin B_{12}	1.4mcg	72.9
Magnesium	24.5mg	8.1	Folic Acid	38.3m	12.8
Potassium	259.9mg	8.7	Starch	4.2g	–
Sodium	111.6mg	9.3	Sugars	34.2g	–
USEFUL FOR: CANCER PREVENTION; HEART DISEASE PREVENTION; STROKE PREVENTION; CHOLESTEROL REDUCTION; DAIRY FOOD ALLERGY DIETS.					

Parsnip and lemon soup (F V 8)

I invented this recipe when planning a dinner party with lemons as the theme of the meal. It proved to be very successful. It is pale lemon in colour, looks very sophisticated and the flavours are delicate.

Preparation Time: 30 minutes
Cooking Time: 45 minutes
Ingredients: Imperial/Metric

2oz/50g	polyunsaturated margarine (unhydrogenated)
1	onion, peeled and sliced
1lb/450g	parsnips, peeled and cubed
8oz/225g	potatoes, washed and cubed
2	garlic cloves, peeled and crushed
2pts/1000ml	vegetable stock
2tsp	saffron or turmeric
	black pepper
1	lemon, juice and zest
5fl oz/150ml	silken tofu, liquidized
	parsley to garnish

Method

1 Melt the margarine in a large saucepan and cook the onion gently until soft, about 5 minutes.
2 Add the parsnips, potatoes and garlic. Cover and cook slowly for 20 minutes – until the vegetables are just soft.
3 Add stock, saffron (or turmeric) and pepper.
4 Bring to the boil and simmer for 10 minutes.
5 Add the lemon rind and juice.
6 Liquidize the soup until smooth.
7 Return to the pan and stir in the tofu.
8 Reheat without boiling.
9 Serve garnished with chopped parsley.

TIP BOX

Try using different herbs and spices in the recipes – it really changes the flavour of the dish.

NUTRITION BOX (per serving)					
	Quantity	% RDA		Quantity	% RDA
Calories	123.8	5.0	Copper	0.1mcg	5.4
Protein	3.1g	5.0	Zinc	0.2mcg	1.5
Total fat	5.8g	7.7	Vitamin A	56.3mg	7.5
made up of:			Vitamin C	15.4mg	51.4
saturated	1.4g	–	Vitamin D	0.5mg	4.9
polyunsat.	3.1g	–	Vitamin E	2.2mg	17.9
mono-unsat.	1.2g	–	Vitamin B_1	0.2mg	24.9
Cholesterol	–	–	Vitamin B_2	0.2mg	17.0
Fibre	2.1g	6.9	Nicotinic Acid	2.5mg	15.1
Iron	2.8mg	27.6	Vitamin B_6	0.1mg	5.5
Calcium	36.1mg	7.2	Vitamin B_{12}	0.7mcg	36.6
Magnesium	18.0mg	6.0	Folic Acid	19.8mg	6.6
Potassium	309.7mg	10.3	Starch	12.1g	–
Sodium	55.9mg	4.7	Sugars	2.9g	–
USEFUL FOR: HYPERTENSION REDUCTION.					

Garlic and Tofu Dip (V 4)

Garlic and tofu blend beautifully together and this makes a nice party dip.
Add some wholemeal breadcrumbs if you prefer a firmer dip.

Preparation Time: 5 minutes
Ingredients: Imperial/Metric
2   garlic cloves, peeled and crushed
2oz/50g   onion, peeled and finely chopped
5fl oz/150ml silken tofu, liquidized
            black pepper

Method

1 Combine all the ingredients well.
2 Serve chilled with raw vegetables.

NUTRITION BOX (per serving)					
	Quantity	% RDA		Quantity	% RDA
Calories	26.8	1.0	Copper	–	–
Protein	2.0g	3.2	Zinc	–	0.5
Total fat	1.0g	1.3	Vitamin A	–	–
made up of:			Vitamin C	1.5mg	5.0
saturated	0.2g	–	Vitamin D	–	–
polyunsat.	0.8g	–	Vitamin E	–	–
mono-unsat.	0.0g	–	Vitamin B_1	0.1mg	5.0
Cholesterol	0.0g	–	Vitamin B_2	–	1.1
Fibre	0.3g	.9	Nicotinic Acid	–	0.4
Iron	0.4mg	4.2	Vitamin B_6	0.1mg	0.6
Calcium	17.3mg	3.5	Vitamin B_{12}	–	–
Magnesium	9.9mg	3.3	Folic Acid	0.2mg	0.1
Potassium	55.1mg	1.8	Starch	1.0g	–
Sodium	1.9mg	.2	Sugars	0.6g	–
USEFUL FOR: HYPERTENSION REDUCTION; DAIRY FOOD ALLERGY DIETS; COELIACS.					

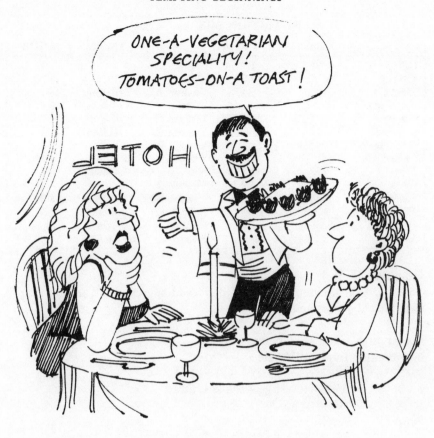

Herb Dip (F 8)

This dip looks very attractive with the chopped green herbs contrasting with the pale yellow of the cheeses.

Preparation Time: 15 minutes
Ingredients: Imperial/Metric
1tbsp	fresh mint, chopped
1tbsp	fresh parsley, chopped
4oz/100g	low fat vegetarian cheese, grated
4oz/100g	low fat vegetarian cottage cheese
4oz/100g	low fat vegetarian soft cheese
2	garlic cloves, peeled and crushed

Method
1 Combine all the ingredients well.
2 Serve chilled piled on top of curly endive leaves.

NUTRITION BOX (per serving)					
	Quantity	% RDA		Quantity	% RDA
Calories	68.0	2.7	Copper	–	.7
Protein	6.7g	10.7	Zinc	0.5mcg	5.3
Total fat	4.1g	5.4	Vitamin A	50.2mg	6.7
made up of:			Vitamin C	3.0mg	10.0
saturated	–	–	Vitamin D	–	.2
polyunsat.	–	–	Vitamin E	0.1mg	1.1
mono-unsat.	–	–	Vitamin B$_1$	–	1.2
Cholesterol	–	–	Vitamin B$_2$	0.1mg	3.9
Fibre	2.3g	7.8	Nicotinic Acid	0.8mg	4.6
Iron	. 2mg	2.0	Vitamin B$_6$	–	.8
Calcium	99.0mg	19.8	Vitamin B$_{12}$	0.1mcg	8.8
Magnesium	4.6mg	1.5	Folic Acid	2.6mg	.9
Potassium	52.2mg	1.7	Starch	1.1g	–
Sodium	123.5mg	10.3	Sugars	–	–

Hummus (F V 4)

This is a light hummus because I don't add any extra oil, so you simply
taste the chick peas and garlic.

Preparation Time: 15 minutes
Ingredients: Imperial/Metric
8oz/225g   chick peas, washed and soaked
2   garlic cloves, peeled and crushed
1tbsp   tahini
1tbsp   lemon juice
              black pepper and low sodium salt
              a little water to aid the liquidizing process

Method

1 Cook the chick peas in water for about 1 hour until tender.
2 Drain the chick peas, reserving 2 tablespoons of the liquid.
3 Place the liquid, lemon juice, tahini, garlic and chick peas into a blender
   and blend until smooth.
4 Season to taste.
5 Serve chilled piled on top of red cabbage or lettuce leaves.

NUTRITION BOX (per serving)					
	Quantity	% RDA		Quantity	% RDA
Calories	251.8	10.1	Copper	0.5mcg	26.9
Protein	12.5g	19.9	Zinc	0.1mcg	1.3
Total fat	3.2g	4.2	Vitamin A	16.8mg	2.3
made up of:			Vitamin C	14.3mg	47.5
saturated	–	–	Vitamin D	.-	–
polyunsat.	–	–	Vitamin E	–	–
mono-unsat.	–	–	Vitamin B$_1$	0.3mg	32.1
Cholesterol	–	–	Vitamin B$_2$	0.1mg	10.2
Fibre	10.3g	34.2	Nicotinic Acid	10.3mg	62.2
Iron	4.0mg	38.7	Vitamin B$_6$	0.1mg	6.4
Calcium	121.6mg	24.3	Vitamin B$_{12}$	–	–
Magnesium	100.5mg	33.5	Folic Acid	56.4mg	18.8
Potassium	631.0mg	21.0	Starch	22.5g	–
Sodium	35.2mg	2.9	Sugars	12.2g	–

USEFUL FOR: HEART DISEASE PREVENTION; HYPERTENSION REDUCTION; CHOLESTEROL REDUCTION; DAIRY FOOD ALLERGY DIETS; COELIACS.

Soft Lentil Pâté (F V 4)
A soft pâté which is popular with our guests. Hot poppy seed rolls (p. 125) or wholemeal toast complement it nicely.

Preparation Time: 20 minutes
Cooking Time: 30 minutes
Ingredients: Imperial/Metric
6oz/175g   continental (small brown) lentils
1oz/25g   polyunsaturated margarine (unhydrogenated)
1   onion, peeled and chopped
6oz/175g   mushrooms, wiped and sliced
1tsp   dried chives
1tsp   dried marjoram
1tsp   lemon juice
     black pepper and low sodium salt

Method
1 Cook the lentils in boiling water until soft, about 20 minutes. Drain well.
2 Meanwhile, melt the margarine and fry the onion until soft, about 5 minutes.
3 Add the mushrooms and fry for 2 minutes, stirring.
4 Add the remaining ingredients and mix well.
5 Pile into ramekin dishes and serve well chilled, garnished with watercress leaves.

NUTRITION BOX (per serving)					
	Quantity	% RDA		Quantity	% RDA
Calories	197	7.9	Copper	28.7mcg	28.7
Protein	11.7g	18.6	Zinc	1.5mcg	14.5
Total fat	6.0g	7.9	Vitamin A	60.6mg	8.1
made up of:			Vitamin C	5.8mg	19.4
saturated	1.4g	–	Vitamin D	0.5mcg	5.0
polyunsat.	2.8g	–	Vitamin E	1.6mg	13.0
mono-unsat.	1.3g	–	Vitamin B$_1$	27.8mg	27.8
Cholesterol	–	–	Vitamin B$_2$	0.3mg	19.8
Fibre	6.9g	22.9	Nicotinic Acid	4.8mg	28.8
Iron	3.9mg	38.2	Vitamin B$_6$	0.4mg	17.8
Calcium	34.1mg	6.8	Vitamin B$_{12}$	0.3mcg	15.6
Magnesium	43.4mg	14.5	Folic Acid	25.4mg	8.5
Potassium	568.8mg	19.0	Starch	22.2g	–
Sodium	74.7mg	6.2	Sugars	3.7g	–

USEFUL FOR: HYPERTENSION REDUCTION; CHOLESTEROL REDUCTION; DAIRY FOOD ALLERGY DIETS; COELIACS.

Mushroom and Seed Pâté (F M 8)

A tasty and versatile pâté: you can change the subtle flavours by using different herbs – rosemary is particularly nice. And use whatever seeds you happen to have, sunflower seeds are always a good standby.

Preparation Time: 30 minutes
Cooking Time: 60 minutes
Temperature: 180°C, 360°F, Gas Mark 4
Ingredients: Imperial/Metric
2oz/50g   polyunsaturated margarine (unhydrogenated)
1   large onion, peeled and chopped
1lb/450g   mushrooms, wiped and sliced
8oz/225g   wholemeal breadcrumbs
4oz/125g   seeds, ground
1   egg white
1tbsp   tahini
1tsp   yeast extract
1tbsp   dried mixed herbs
    black pepper and low sodium salt

Method
1 Grease and line a 450g (1lb) loaf tin.
2 Melt the margarine and fry the onion for 5 minutes until soft.
3 Add the mushrooms and cook until the liquid evaporates.
4 Liquidize the mixture.
5 Add all the remaining ingredients and mix well.
6 Pour the mixture into the prepared tin.

7 Cover with greased foil and cook for about 1 hour, in a preheated oven.
8 Allow to cool for at least 10 minutes before turning out.

NUTRITION BOX (per serving)					
	Quantity	% RDA		Quantity	% RDA
Calories	177.4	7.1	Copper	0.5mcg	22.8
Protein	3.7g	5.9	Zinc	0.6mcg	6.4
Total fat	6.3g	8.5	Vitamin A	56.2mg	7.5
made up of:			Vitamin C	3.9mg	13.1
saturated	1.5g	–	Vitamin D	0.5mcg	4.9
polyunsat.	3.2g	–	Vitamin E	6.4mg	53.8
mono-unsat.	1.3g	–	Vitamin B_1	0.4mg	44.4
Cholesterol	–	–	Vitamin B_2	0.3mg	20.1
Fibre	3.3g	11.1	Nicotinic Acid	3.2mg	19.3
Iron	2.5mg	23.8	Vitamin B_6	0.1mg	6.1
Calcium	34.9mg	7.0	Vitamin B_{12}	0.5mcg	23.9
Magnesium	41.4mg	13.8	Folic Acid	24.2mg	8.1
Potassium	505.0mg	16.8	Starch	11.2g	–
Sodium	209.4mg	17.4	Sugars	1.3g	–
USEFUL FOR: MILK ALLERGY DIETS.					

Vegetable Pâté (F M 8)

This pâté is pale green in colour and has a lovely and creamy texture.

Preparation Time: 45 minutes
Cooking Time: 30 minutes
Temperature: 180°C, 350°F, Gas Mark 4
Ingredients: Imperial/Metric
2lb/1000g courgettes, washed and grated
1tbsp sea salt
2oz/50g polyunsaturated margarine (unhydrogenated)
1 onion, peeled and chopped
3 garlic cloves, peeled and crushed
4 egg whites, whisked until stiff
2tsp mustard
2tbsp fresh herbs, chopped
10fl oz/250ml silken tofu, liquidized
4oz/100g broccoli, washed and lightly steamed
 pinch cayenne pepper
 black pepper and low sodium salt

Method

1 Grease and line a 900g (2lb) loaf tin.
2 Place the courgettes in a colander and sprinkle with the salt. Leave to drain for 30 minutes. Rinse under cold running water and then leave to drain again.

3   Melt the margarine and fry the onion and garlic for 5 minutes. Add the courgettes and cook for 10 minutes. Stir well.

4   Remove from the heat and cool slightly.

5   Add the courgette mixture, herbs, mustard and the seasoning to the tofu.

6   Carefully fold in the egg whites.

7   Pour half the courgette mixture into the prepared tin.

8   Place the broccoli in a layer over the courgettes.

9   Pour over the remaining courgette mixture.

10   Cover the tin with foil and stand in a roasting tin which has 5 cm (2 in) of cold water in it.

11   Cook in a preheated oven for 1 hour 15 minutes.

12   Allow to cool for at least 10 minutes before turning out of the tin. Chill in tin. Serve garnished with tomato slices and watercress leaves.

> ### TIP BOX
>
> You can make the pâté look and taste different by layering it. Alternate the pâté with layers of tomatoes, mushrooms or low fat cheeses.

NUTRITION BOX (per serving)

	Quantity	% RDA		Quantity	% RDA
Calories	121.8	4.9	Copper	–	1.5
Protein	4.2g	6.6	Zinc	0.1mcg	0.9
Total fat	6.6g	8.8	Vitamin A	207.5mg	27.7
made up of:			Vitamin C	28.1mg	93.5
saturated	1.4g	–	Vitamin D	0.5mcg	4.9
polyunsat.	3.4g	–	Vitamin E	1.7mg	14.2
mono-unsat.	1.3g	–	Vitamin B_1	0.1mg	11.3
Cholesterol	–	–	Vitamin B_2	0.2mg	10.8
Fibre	3.2g	10.6	Nicotinic Acid	0.8mg	4.6
Iron	3.5mg	34.2	Vitamin B_6	–	2.1
Calcium	66.0mg	13.2	Vitamin B_{12}	0.3mcg	15.6
Magnesium	18.3mg	6.1	Folic Acid	73.9mg	24.6
Potassium	341.7mg	11.4	Starch	0.5g	–
Sodium	54.8mg	4.6	Sugars	7.1g	–

USEFUL FOR: CANCER PREVENTION; HEART DISEASE PREVENTION; STROKE PREVENTION; CHOLESTEROL REDUCTION; HYPERTENSION REDUCTION; MILK ALLERGY DIETS; COELIACS.

> ### TIP BOX
>
> Watercress is the same species as the nasturtium that is grown commonly in gardens. The flowers and leaves of this plant are edible and look very attractive in salads or as garnishes.

Tomato Moulds (V 4)

These bright little moulds look mouthwatering with the different vegetables and seeds suspended in the bright red of the tomato 'jelly'. I use 'Gelozone' as the setting agent instead of the traditional gelatine which contains animal extracts.

Preparation Time: 20 minutes
Cooking Time: 5 minutes
Setting Time: 30 minutes
Ingredients: Imperial/Metric

¼pt/150ml	tomato juice
1tsp	Gelozone
1	stick celery, washed and chopped
1oz/25g	onion, grated
2oz/50g	sunflower seeds
1oz/25g	watercress, washed and chopped
1tbsp	fresh mint, washed and chopped
	black pepper

Method

1 Pour the tomato juice into a saucepan and heat gently.
2 Sprinkle on the Gelozone and whisk in until well blended.
3 Stir and continue to heat until the juice begins to steam – do not allow to boil.
4 Remove from the heat and add all the remaining ingredients – stirring well.
5 Spoon the mixture into individual moulds (I use small, round plastic microwave moulds) and leave to set in the fridge for about 30 minutes.
6 Turn out onto a serving plate and garnish.

NUTRITION BOX (per serving)					
	Quantity	% RDA		Quantity	% RDA
Calories	42.6	1.7	Copper	–	0.7
Protein	.6g	.5	Zinc	0.1mcg	0.5
Total fat	–	–	Vitamin A	25.9mg	3.5
made up of:			Vitamin C	4.7mg	15.6
saturated	–	–	Vitamin D	–	–
polyunsat.	–	–	Vitamin E	3.9mg	32.8
mono-unsat.	–	–	Vitamin B_1	0.3mg	26.2
Cholesterol	–	–	Vitamin B_2	0.04mg	2.8
Fibre	0.3g	1.0	Nicotinic Acid	0.1mg	0.7
Iron	1.0mg	10.2	Vitamin B_6	0.01mg	0.7
Calcium	31.4mg	6.3	Vitamin B_{12}	–	–
Magnesium	6.6mg	2.2	Folic Acid	12.7mg	4.2
Potassium	157.1mg	5.2	Starch	1.3g	–
Sodium	5.1mg	.4	Sugars	0.3g	–
USEFUL FOR: HYPERTENSION REDUCTION; DAIRY FOOD ALLERGY DIETS; COELIACS.					

Melon, Cheese and Ginger Refresher (8)

Wonderfully simple to make and delicious to eat. The sweet, juicy melon combines beautifully with the textures of the ginger and the apple.

Preparation Time: 10 minutes
Ingredients: Imperial/Metric
½   melon, chopped
8oz/250g   low fat cottage cheese
1oz/25g   preserved ginger, chopped finely
1   red apple, washed well and chopped
            black pepper
8   chicory leaves
8   sprigs fresh mint
            paprika pepper

Method

1   Combine the first five ingredients together.
2   Pile into tall elegant glasses and garnish with the chicory leaves and mint sprigs.
3   Sprinkle a little paprika pepper on top of each one.

NUTRITION BOX (per serving)					
	Quantity	% RDA		Quantity	% RDA
Calories	57.6	2.3	Copper	0.03mcg	1.8
Protein	4.0g	6.3	Zinc	0.1mcg	0.7
Total fat	2.7g	3.6	Vitamin A	9.1mg	1.2
made up of:			Vitamin C	14.5mg	48.3
saturated	–	–	Vitamin D	–	–
polyunsat.	–	–	Vitamin E	0.1mg	0.8
mono-unsat.	–	–	Vitamin B_1	0.03mg	3.1
Cholesterol	–	–	Vitamin B_2	–	–
Fibre	3.5g	11.6	Nicotinic Acid	0.3mg	1.7
Iron	0.2mg	1.5	Vitamin B_6	0.04mg	4.0
Calcium	8.1mg	1.6	Vitamin B_{12}	–	–
Magnesium	7.3mg	2.4	Folic Acid	17.2mg	5.8
Potassium	136.9mg	4.6	Starch	0.8g	–
Sodium	11.0mg	.9	Sugars	3.7g	–
USEFUL FOR: HYPERTENSION REDUCTION; COELIACS.					

TIP BOX

If you prefer your pâte to have a smoother consistency, just liquidize for a little longer.

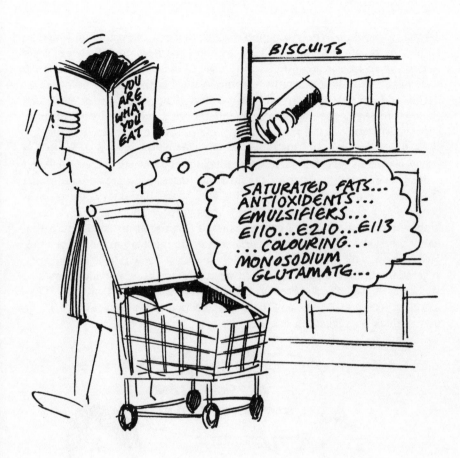

6
LIFE AFTER MEAT AND TWO VEG'

To many people a vegetarian meal would, at best, consist of an omelette with chips or a cheese salad. These are the two alternatives I always seem to have when we eat in a pub. And neither of these is particularly good for your health. So often a healthy vegetarian meal is thought to be tasteless, boring and unappetizing. I wish I had collected a pound coin for each time these words have been spoken to me at the very suggestion of vegetarian cuisine. In some cases, I must admit, these phrases may be well justified.

Last year we had an Australian couple staying at our guest house – a lovely couple in their late fifties. Upon being asked whether they preferred vegetarian or traditional cuisine the husband very eagerly stressed traditional food, causing a frown to appear on his wife's face. Traditional cuisine was considered a treat for him as he had heart trouble and was vegetarian at home for medical reasons. I expressed great surprise at his change in eating habits when abroad. But more surprising was the explanation for this change. Not being a cook himself he unwillingly ate what his wife considered to be vegetarian cuisine – a plate of cooked vegetables served with boiled potatoes! We soon showed them there was more to vegetarian food than that! They left us to return to Australia with a good selection of my recipes and a whole new outlook on vegetarian cuisine.

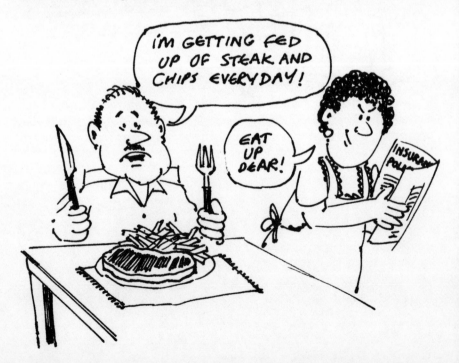

The basis of traditional main course meals is either red meat, poultry or fish and these are easy to replace with pulses, legumes, grains, seeds and vegetables. There is no point, from the health angle, in replacing the high fat meats in a recipe with other high fat ingredients such as cheese and eggs. This defeats the object. So being vegetarian is not synonymous with eating a healthy diet as many people believe. My recipes rely heavily on low fat ingredients, but that does not mean the meals are short on taste.

The main course is the centrepiece of any meal and it is well worth a little extra effort to present it with style and imagination. The appearance of a dish makes such a difference. Just spend a few minutes trying to imagine what the meal will look like on the plate, thinking particularly of colours, textures and shapes. Arrange the food on the plate rather than simply spooning piles of it anywhere. It only takes a minute and yet it makes such a big difference to the appearance of the meal and, as a result, makes it more appetizing. Vegetarian food is colourful and exciting and this should be reflected in its presentation.

Common problems

The main problem people seem to encounter when thinking of vegetarian main courses is what to actually serve. There is much more to vegetarian cuisine than simply knocking the meat off the plate. Cooking healthily involves thinking about food in a different way. The method of cooking and the ingredients used need to be reassessed. Initially it may be difficult to imagine a main course without meat but once you realize that vegetables need not be relegated to being a mere accompaniment to meat an exciting new concept in food opens up. The recipes in this chapter will give you some idea of the variety and scope available and, hopefully, give you ideas to try for yourself.

The time element seems to be another problem for many people – or, rather, they think it is. Initially you will probably find that cooking vegetarian takes a little longer than cooking traditional. However, in most cases, this is because you are attempting something new which involves quite a bit of thought and not because it is vegetarian. It is not just a case of switching into automatic pilot any more for choosing your ingredients and cooking them – you now have to concentrate and this takes both time and effort. Once you become familiar with the processes involved you will find that it takes no longer to cook vegetarian – in fact it can be much quicker. For one thing there is no meat to contend with, and that accounts for a large slice of the cooking time of a dish. Fresh vegetables, fruit, pulses and legumes are used instead. And although soaking is required for some legumes, such as dried beans, this only takes a minute to prepare and pulses, such as lentils, need no soaking at all. If you're in a hurry then tinned legumes are available which are quite good but most do contain added salt – read the labels. The use of a pressure cooker will also cut down the cooking time involved.

People often tell me that when they have tried to cook a vegetarian meal the result is bland and tasteless. One of the main reasons is overcooking the vegetables as you lose most of their flavour, not to mention their texture. Another cause, particularly if salt is not used, is the seasoning. Herbs and spices are an important part of any cooking but they are of paramount importance in vegetarian cuisine. Experiment with the many herbs and spices available and you will soon see that no dish need be tasteless.

Conversion recipes

Transforming traditional main course meals into healthy ones is very easy once you know some of the ground rules. The thing to remember is that we are aiming to reduce the amount of salt, sugar and fat, particularly saturated fat, in our diet and to increase the amount of fibre. Translating this information into everyday eating habits means that meats are replaced with pulses, legumes, grains and vegetables and that high fat dairy products are replaced with low fat alternatives. This not only cuts down on the amount of fat consumed but also increases our fibre intake. The amount of salt used in cooking and at the table can be reduced, even eliminated, by seasoning with herbs, spices and fruit zests. It is surprising how quickly your tastebuds will adapt to eating less salt.

If you feel that you cannot make these changes all at once then do it gradually – perhaps reducing the meat content in a recipe by half and using lentils instead. It is far better to do this than not to make any change to your diet at all. You will probably find that as you become accustomed to eating less meat you will actually prefer eating healthy vegetarian meals.

I have chosen three recipes to convert into healthier alternatives and this will give you some idea of the process involved.

TRADITIONAL RECIPE	**CONVERSION RECIPE**
Lasagne	**Lasagne**
½ packet lasagne verde	½ packet wholewheat lasagne
1 large tin minced beef	1lb/500g vegetables
1tbsp tomato purée	1tbs tomato purée (sugar and salt free)
garlic salt	1 garlic clove
black pepper	black pepper
½pt/250ml single cream	½pt/250ml silken tofu
2oz/50g Cheddar cheese	2oz/50g low fat vegetarian cheese
Lamb with Dumplings	**Casserole with Dumplings**
1½lb/675g lamb	8oz/225g dried chick peas
	8oz/225g dried red kidney beans
2tbsp seasoned flour	
1tbsp butter	1tbsp extra virgin olive oil
2 onions	2 onions
4oz peas	4oz peas
½pt/250ml water	½pt/250ml vegetable stock
1 beef stock cube	
1lb/500g carrots	1lb/500g carrots

Dumplings:
4oz/125g self raising flour

2oz/50g suet
1tbsp mixed herbs
black pepper
cold water

French Onion Tart

8oz/225g shortcrust pastry
1lb/500g onion
2oz/50g butter
1tsp salt

2 eggs
3fl oz/75ml single cream
3oz/75g Cheddar cheese

Dumplings:
4oz/125g plain wholemeal flour
1tsp low sodium baking powder
2oz/50g polyunsaturated margarine
1tbsp mixed herbs
black pepper
cold water

French Onion Tart

8oz/225g low fat pastry
1lb/500g onion
2oz/50g extra virgin olive oil
½tsp nutmeg
½tsp tarragon
2 egg whites
3fl oz/75ml silken tofu
3oz/75g low fat vegetarian cheese

Low Fat Pastry (F)

This pastry cuts down on the need for fat by using yeast to 'lighten' it. The addition of the yeast also makes the pastry easier to handle than the 'normal' wholemeal variety.

Preparation Time: 25 minutes
Ingredients: Imperial/Metric

5oz/175g	plain wholemeal flour
1oz/25g	soya flour
½tsp	dried yeast, easy blend
	pinch of vitamin C powder
1	egg white, lightly beaten
1fl oz/25ml	sesame oil, cold pressed
6tsp	warm water

Method

1 Mix the flours, yeast and vitamin C in a bowl and add the egg white.
2 Mix the oil and warm water together and add to the bowl.
3 Form the dough into a ball and knead on a lightly floured work surface for about 6 or 7 minutes.
4 Leave the dough to rest in a lightly oiled polythene bag until required.

NUTRITION BOX (per serving)					
	Quantity	% RDA		Quantity	% RDA
Calories	229	9.2	Copper	0.2mcg	11.9
Protein	8.5g	13.6	Zinc	1.4mcg	14.1
Total fat	8.6g	11.5	Vitamin A	–	–
made up of:			Vitamin C	–	–
saturated	1.2g	–	Vitamin D	–	–
polyunsat.	1.9g	–	Vitamin E	0.8mg	6.2
mono-unsat.	4.7g	–	Vitamin B$_1$	0.3mg	27.7
Cholesterol	–	–	Vitamin B$_2$	0.1mg	7.2
Fibre	4.6g	15.5	Nicotinic Acid	2.3mg	13.9
Iron	2.4mg	23.6	Vitamin B$_6$	0.3mg	14.0
Calcium	29.4mg	5.9	Vitamin B$_{12}$	–	–
Magnesium	79.1mg	26.4	Folic Acid	74.9mg	25.0
Potassium	286.2mg	9.5	Starch	28.6g	–
Sodium	2.0mg	0.2	Sugars	158.2g	–
USEFUL FOR: MILK ALLERGY DIETS; HYPERTENSION REDUCTION.					

Spiced Parcels (F V 8)

These delicious, fragrantly spiced parcels are delicious eaten hot or cold – especially with some garlic and tofu dip (p. 48).

Preparation Time: 40 minutes
Cooking Time: 30 minutes
Temperature: 200°C, 400°F, Gas Mark 6
Ingredients: Imperial/Metric

2tbsp	extra virgin olive oil
2tsp	cumin seeds
1tsp	maram gasala
1tsp	ground coriander
4oz/100g	potatoes, washed and diced
4oz/100g	onion, peeled and diced
2	garlic cloves, peeled and crushed
4oz/100g	spinach, washed
4oz/100g	chick peas, washed, soaked and cooked
1tbsp	tahini
	black pepper
1 quantity	low fat pastry (see p. 61)

Method

1 Heat the oil in a medium-sized saucepan and add the cumin seeds and spices. Cook for 2 minutes.
2 Add the diced potato, onions and garlic and gently cook for about 10 minutes.

3 Add the spinach and cook for 4 minutes.
4 Add the chick peas, tahini and pepper. Cook for 2 minutes, stirring.
5 Roll out the pastry into a rectangle measuring 30 × 60 cm (12 × 24in) and divide into eight 15cm (6in) squares.
6 Divide the spiced mixture equally between the pastry squares, spreading it diagonally across half the surface of the pastry.
7 Dampen the edges of the pastry with a little water and fold the pastry over to form a triangle shape. Press the pastry edges together firmly to seal the parcels.
8 Place the parcels on a lightly greased baking tray and cook in a preheated oven for about 30 minutes until they are golden brown and heated through.

NUTRITION BOX (per serving)					
	Quantity	% RDA		Quantity	% RDA
Calories	143	5.7	Copper	0.3mcg	15.1
Protein	7.0g	7.0	Zinc	0.2mcg	2.1
Total fat	1.6g	2.1	Vitamin A	307.5mg	41.0
made up of:			Vitamin C	14.1mg	47.1
saturated	0.02g	–	Vitamin D	–	–
polyunsat.	0.1g	–	Vitamin E	0.5mg	4.4
mono-unsat.	–	–	Vitamin B_1	0.2mg	17.9
Cholesterol	–	–	Vitamin B_2	0.1mg	6.7
Fibre	5.9g	19.7	Nicotinic Acid	1.9mg	11.5
Iron	2.8mg	27.2	Vitamin B_6	0.1mg	5.8
Calcium	194.4mg	38.9	Vitamin B_{12}	–	–
Magnesium	60.8mg	20.3	Folic Acid	62.8mg	20.9
Potassium	454.0mg	15.1	Starch	15.9g	–
Sodium	43.9mg	3.7	Sugars	4.2g	–
USEFUL FOR: CANCER PREVENTION; HEART DISEASE PREVENTION; MILK ALLERGY DIETS; HYPERTENSION REDUCTION; CHOLESTEROL REDUCTION.					

Stuffed Aubergines (F V 4)
Aubergines lend themselves to almost any kind of tasty stuffing.

Preparation Time: 80 minutes
Cooking Time: 40 minutes
Temperature: 200°C, 400°F, Gas Mark 6
Ingredients: Imperial/Metric
2   large aubergines
1oz/25g   polyunsaturated margarine (unhydrogenated)
1   large onion, peeled and chopped
4oz/100g   raisins
5oz/150g   wholemeal breadcrumbs
6oz/175g   mushrooms, wiped and sliced

2oz/50g	sunflower seeds, roasted, roughly chopped
2tbsp	fresh parsley, chopped finely
1tsp	dried marjoram
1tsp	ground coriander
1tbsp	tahini
2 fl oz/50ml	vegetable stock
1tbsp	orange (well scrubbed) zest
1tbsp	pumpkin seeds
	black pepper

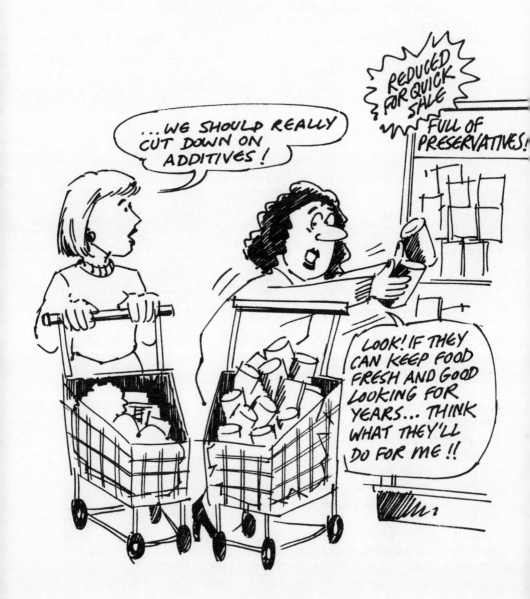

Method

1 Wash the aubergines and cut in half lengthways. Carefully scoop out the flesh from each aubergine. Leave about a 6mm (¼ inch) thickness to form the 'shell'.
2 Dice the flesh and place in a colander. Sprinkle with salt and shake to make sure that all the pieces have salt on them. Sprinkle the aubergine shells with salt also. Leave for 1 hour.
3 Wash under running water and drain. This process rids the aubergines of their bitter juices.
4 Melt the margarine and add the onion. Fry for 5 minutes until soft but not brown.
5 Add the chopped aubergine and cook for a further 10 minutes.
6 Transfer to a bowl and add all the remaining ingredients. Mix well.
7 Pile the mixture into the aubergine shells and place in an ovenproof dish and cook in a preheated oven until the mixture is beginning to crisp up and go a golden brown. Serve hot with a crisp salad.

TIP BOX

To keep stuffed vegetables upright during cooking pack crinkled foil around them.

NUTRITION BOX (per serving)					
	Quantity	% RDA		Quantity	% RDA
Calories	514	20.6	Copper	0.62mcg	31.3
Protein	6.8g	10.9	Zinc	0.91mcg	9.1
Total fat	6.6g	8.7	Vitamin A	98.7mg	13.2
made up of:			Vitamin C	22.0mg	73.3
saturated	1.5g	–	Vitamin D	0.49mcg	4.9
polyunsat.	3.3g	–	Vitamin E	7.5mg	62.6
mono-unsat.	1.2g	–	Vitamin B_1	0.75mg	75.6
Cholesterol	–	–	Vitamin B_2	0.49mg	34.1
Fibre	9.8g	32.5	Nicotinic Acid	5.7mg	34.5
Iron	57.5mg	57.5	Vitamin B_6	0.35mg	17.7
Calcium	92.7mg	18.5	Vitamin B_{12}	0.64mcg	32.3
Magnesium	79.6mg	26.5	Folic Acid	55.8mg	18.6
Potassium	38.5mg	38.5	Starch	15.3g	
Sodium	280.9mg	23.4	Sugars	24.2g	–
USEFUL FOR: CANCER PREVENTION; HEART DISEASE PREVENTION; STROKE PREVENTION; DAIRY FOOD ALLERGY DIETS; CHOLESTEROL REDUCTION.					

Carrot and Mushroom Roulade (F 4)

A delicious and attractive main course which will impress anyone – especially when you tell them it doesn't contain egg yolks. Like most of my recipes, this was developed for Richard who loves soufflé-type dishes but can't eat traditional ones because of the egg yolks. You can adapt the recipe by using a different vegetable, such as spinach, and low fat soft cheese for the filling.

Preparation Time: 45 minutes
Cooking Time: 30 minutes
Temperature: 200°C, 400°F, Gas Mark 6
Ingredients: Imperial/Metric

2oz/50g	polyunsaturated margarine (unhydrogerated)
3oz/75g	wholemeal or granary flour
10fl oz/250ml	soya milk (sugar free)
1lb/450g	carrots, grated
2tbsp	tahini
2tsp	marjoram
	black pepper
2	egg whites
6fl oz/175ml	silken tofu, liquidized
8oz/225g	mushrooms, wiped and chopped
	nutmeg, freshly grated
3oz/75g	sunflower seeds, roasted
2oz/50g	wholemeal breadcrumbs
	low sodium salt

Method

1 Oil and line a 28cm (11in) Swiss roll tin.
2 Melt margarine in a pan and add 2oz of the flour. Cook for 1 minute, stirring.
3 Remove pan from heat and add the milk gradually, stirring all the time. Bring to the boil and then simmer for about 5 minutes until the sauce thickens.
4 Remove from the heat and add the carrots, tahini, marjoram and pepper.
5 Whisk egg whites until stiff and carefully fold into the mixture. Spoon into the prepared tin, level, and cook for about 20 minutes until well risen and golden brown.
6 Meanwhile, place tofu in a saucepan and bring gently to the boil, add the remaining flour and stir. Simmer until the sauce thickens.
7 Add the mushrooms and simmer very gently for 5 minutes. Remove from the heat and add the nutmeg, sunflower seeds and pepper. Leave to cool.
8 When the roulade is cooked turn it out onto a sheet of greaseproof paper sprinkled with breadcrumbs. Remove the greaseproof lining paper.

9 Make a shallow cut about ½" (1cm) from one of the short ends of the roulade. This will make the rolling up easier.

10 Spoon the mushroom mixture onto the roulade but do not cover the little cut. Then carefully roll the roulade up like a Swiss roll.

11 Gently ease the roulade back towards the centre of the greaseproof paper, then, holding the edges of the greaseproof paper, lift the roulade back onto the Swiss roll tin and return to the oven for 10 minutes to heat through. Slice and serve hot.

NUTRITION BOX (per serving)					
	Quantity	% RDA		Quantity	% RDA
Calories	353	14.2	Copper	0.56mcg	27.9
Protein	9.5g	15.2	Zinc	1.2mcg	12.2
Total fat	13.9g	18.6	Vitamin A	2362.5mg	315.0
made up of:			Vitamin C	6.2mg	20.6
saturated	3.0g	–	Vitamin D	0.98mcg	9.8
polyunsat.	7.9g	–	Vitamin E	9.7mg	80.9
mono-unsat.	2.5g	–	Vitamin B_1	0.66mg	66.5
Cholesterol	–	–	Vitamin B_2	0.36mg	24.6
Fibre	7.4g	24.7	Nicotinic acid	3.8mg	23.2
Iron	4.4mg	43.1	Vitamin B_6	0.64mg	32.2
Calcium	136.6mg	27.3	Vitamin B_{12}	0.62mcg	32.5
Magnesium	81.0mg	27.0	Folic acid	37.5mg	12.5
Potassium	673.9mg	22.4	Starch	17.0g	–
Sodium	232.6mg	19.4	Sugars	72.5g	–

USEFUL FOR: CANCER PREVENTION; HEART DISEASE PREVENTION; STROKE PREVENTION; MILK ALLERGY DIETS; HYPERTENSION REDUCTION; CHOLESTEROL REDUCTION.

TIP BOX

Tofu is very versatile and can be used for savoury and sweet dishes alike. The natural flavour of tofu is extremely bland – it takes on the flavours you mix with it.

Chick Pea Moussaka (F 8)

This recipe comes with the recommendation of a great friend – a confirmed meat eater!

Preparation Time: 45 minutes
Cooking Time: 50 minutes
Temperature: 190°C, 375°F, Gas Mark 5
Ingredients: Imperial/Metric

2tbsp	sesame oil, cold pressed
2	aubergines, sliced 6mm (¼in) thick
1oz/25g	polyunsaturated margarine (unhydrogenated)
1	onion, peeled and chopped
3	garlic cloves, peeled and crushed
6oz/175g	mushrooms, wiped and sliced
2tbsp	wholemeal flour
10fl oz/250ml	soya milk (sugar free)
5fl oz/150ml	vegetable stock
14oz/400g	chick peas, cooked
1	lemon (well washed) zest
	black pepper

Topping:

10fl oz/250ml	plain, unsweetened yogurt
2	egg whites
2oz/50g	low fat vegetarian cheese
2oz/50g	low fat soft cheese

Method

1 Brush two baking sheets with a little oil. Arrange the aubergine slices in single layers on the baking sheet and brush with the remaining oil. Bake in the preheated oven for about 20 minutes until the aubergines are soft.
2 Meanwhile melt the margarine in a saucepan and add the onion. Fry gently for about 5 minutes.
3 Add the garlic and cook for one minute.
4 Add the mushrooms and fry for a further 2 minutes.
5 Stir in the flour and cook for 1 minute.
6 Add the soya milk and stock gradually, stirring all the time. Bring to the boil and simmer for 3 minutes.
7 Stir in the chick peas, lemon rind and pepper. Place half this mixture in an ovenproof dish and cover with half the aubergines. Repeat these layers.
8 Beat the yogurt with the egg whites and half the grated cheese. Add the soft cheese in small bits. Pour the cheese mixture onto the aubergines and sprinkle on the remaining grated cheese.

9 Place in the oven and cook until the topping is golden brown.
10 Serve hot with a large mixed salad.

NUTRITION BOX (per serving)					
	Quantity	% RDA		Quantity	% RDA
Calories	281	11.3	Copper	0.63mcg	31.4
Protein	15.5g	24.7	Zinc	0.45mcg	4.5
Total fat	10.9g	14.5	Vitamin A	92.3mg	12.3
made up of:			Vitamin C	12.7mg	42.3
saturated	1.1g	–	Vitamin D	0.26mcg	2.6
polyunsat.	2.3g	–	Vitamin E	1.1mg	8.9
mono-unsat.	3.0g	–	Vitamin B$_1$	0.35mg	35.5
Cholesterol	–	–	Vitamin B$_2$	0.24mg	16.6
Fibre	11.2g	37.3	Nicotinic Acid	4.3mg	26.0
Iron	4.5mg	43.6	Vitamin B$_6$	0.37mg	15.9
Calcium	168.8mg	33.7	Vitamin B$_{12}$	0.24mcg	12.2
Magnesium	105.4mg	35.1	Folic Acid	70.7mg	23.6
Potassium	766.7mg	25.6	Starch	22.8g	–
Sodium	116.1mg	9.7	Sugars	19.6g	–

USEFUL FOR: HEART DISEASE PREVENTION; CHOLESTEROL
REDUCTION; HYPERTENSION REDUCTION.

TIP BOX

Don't cook pulses and legumes in the
water they were soaked in. It could
give you flatulence!

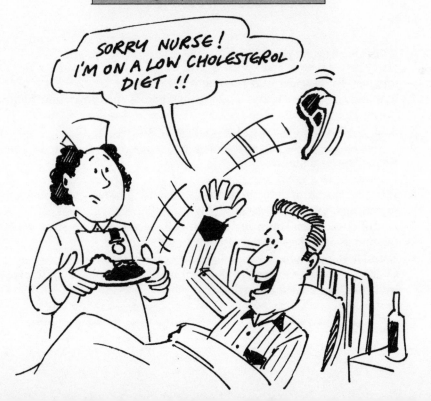

Courgette with Caraway Dumplings (F 4)

Richard loves dumplings but cannot eat the traditional ones because of the suet in them, so I invented this recipe for him. The caraway seeds give the dumplings a very distinctive flavour, although fennel seeds could also be used.

Preparation Time: 45 minutes
Cooking Time: 40 minutes
Temperature: 180°C, 350°F, Gas Mark 4
Ingredients: Imperial/Metric

8oz/225g	courgettes, washed
3oz/75g	polyunsaturated margarine (unhydrogenated)
8oz/225g	baby onions peeled – or large ones sliced
1lb/450g	carrots, washed and sliced
2tbsp	paprika
2tbsp	potato flour
1pt/500ml	vegetable stock
2tsp	dried rosemary
	black pepper

Dumplings

8oz/225g	wholemeal flour
4tsp	baking powder – low sodium
4oz/100g	polyunsaturated margarine (unhydrogenated)
2tsp	caraway seeds
5fl oz/150ml	silken tofu, liquidized
1tbsp	lemon, juice and zest (well scrubbed)
5tbsp	water

Method

1 Slice the courgettes and sprinkle with salt. Leave in a colander for 30 minutes. Rinse under cold running water. Drain.
2 Melt the margarine and fry the courgettes, onions and carrots until lightly browned.
3 Add paprika and flour. Fry for 2 minutes, stirring.
4 Gradually stir in the stock, rosemary and pepper. Bring to the boil and simmer for 5 minutes.
5 Place in an ovenproof dish.
6 Rub the margarine into the flour and baking powder. Add remaining ingredients, except the water.
7 Add the water and form into a firm ball. Divide into 16 small round dumplings and place on top of the courgette mixture.
8 Sprinkle the dumplings with a few extra caraway seeds.
9 Cook in a preheated oven for about 40 minutes until the dumplings are well risen and golden brown.

NUTRITION BOX (per serving)					
	Quantity	% RDA		Quantity	% RDA
Calories	647	25.9	Copper	0.31mcg	15.2
Protein	10.1g	16.1	Zinc	1.9mcg	19.1
Total fat	49.3g	65.8	Vitamin A	1631.2mg	217.5
made up of:			Vitamin C	7.3mg	24.4
saturated	12.1g	–	Vitamin D	4.3mcg	44.4
polyunsat.	25.5g	–	Vitamin E	14.9mg	124.3
mono-unsat.	11.2g	–	Vitamin B_1	0.3mg	34.1
Cholesterol	–	–	Vitamin B_2	0.1mg	7.1
Fibre	7.6g	25.3	Nicotinic acid	1.9mg	11.6
Iron	3.1mg	30.6	Vitamin B_6	0.4mg	19.4
Calcium	72.9mg	14.6	Vitamin B_{12}	2.8mcg	140.6
Magnesium	95.2mg	31.8	Folic acid	36.6mg	12.2
Potassium	353.8mg	11.8	Starch	35.8g	–
Sodium	485.4mg	40.5	Sugars	207.8g	–

USEFUL FOR: CANCER PREVENTION; HEART DISEASE PREVENTION; STROKE PREVENTION; DAIRY FOOD ALLERGY DIETS.

TIP BOX

Try using herbs, spices and fruit zest as seasoning instead of salt, it's healthier and helps ring the changes.

Festive Loaf (F 4)

I invented this recipe mid morning one Christmas Day and, yes, it was for our Christmas dinner. Thank goodness it worked! I wanted to capture the taste of traditional Christmas fare and so the sage and cranberries are of paramount importance to this dish – hence the name.

Preparation Time: 90 minutes
Cooking Time: 90 minutes
Temperature: 180°C, 350°F, Gas Mark 4
Ingredients: Imperial/Metric
Mushroom and sage layer

2tbsp	extra virgin olive oil
1	onion, peeled and chopped
6oz/175g	mushrooms, wiped and sliced
2oz/50g	wholemeal breadcrumbs
2tsp	dried sage
1tbsp	sunflower seeds, roasted
1tbsp	tahini
1tbsp	soya milk

71

black pepper and low sodium salt

Cranberry and apricot layer

1tbsp	extra virgin olive oil
1	onion, peeled and chopped
4oz/100g	cranberries, washed
2oz/50g	wholemeal breadcrumbs
2oz/50g	sunflower seeds, roasted and ground
2oz/50g	dried apricots, soaked and chopped (unsulphurated)
1tbsp	tahini
1tbsp	soya milk
	black pepper and low sodium salt

Split pea layer

1tbsp	extra virgin olive oil
1	onion, peeled and chopped
6oz/175g	yellow split peas, washed, soaked and cooked
1	egg white
	black pepper and low sodium salt

Method

1 Grease and line a 900g (2lb) loaf tin.
2 *Mushroom layer*. Heat the oil and fry the onion until soft but not browned, about 5 minutes. Add the mushrooms and fry for 3 minutes.
3 In a bowl mix in all the remaining ingredients and put to one side.
4 *Cranberry layer*. Heat the oil and fry the onion until soft.
5 In a bowl mix in all the remaining ingredients and put to one side.
6 *Split pea layer*. Heat the oil and fry the onion until soft and add to the split peas.
7 Beat the egg and add to the mixture. Season to taste.
8 Place the mushroom mixture in the base of the tin, pressing it down firmly with the back of a spoon.
9 Then add the cranberry layer, pressing down very firmly.
10 Add the split pea layer and press down firmly. Cover with greased foil and bake in a preheated oven for 1 hour 30 minutes. Allow to cool for at least 10 minutes before turning out of the tin. This is lovely served, hot or cold, with a cranberry sauce.

NUTRITION BOX (per serving)					
	Quantity	% RDA		Quantity	% RDA
Calories	512	20.5	Copper	0.76mcg	38.2
Protein	14.5g	23.1	Zinc	2.3mcg	22.8
Total fat	20.4g	27.2	Vitamin A	45.8mg	6.1
made up of:			Vitamin C	21.2mg	70.6
saturated	3.0g	–	Vitamin D	–	–
polyunsat.	2.7g	–	Vitamin E	6.4mg	53.4
mono-unsat.	14.6g	–	Vitamin B_1	0.84mg	84.3
Cholesterol	–	–	Vitamin B_2	0.42mg	29.3
Fibre	14.4g	48.1	Nicotinic Acid	6.3mg	38.4
Iron	5.4mg	52.8	Vitamin B_6	0.38mg	19.2
Calcium	126.4mg	25.3	Vitamin B_{12}	–	–
Magnesium	107.8mg	35.9	Folic Acid	35.3mg	11.7
Potassium	1236.7mg	41.2	Starch	30.7g	–
Sodium	177.8mg	14.8	Sugars	14.2g	–

USEFUL FOR: CANCER PREVENTION; HEART DISEASE
PREVENTION; STROKE PREVENTION; MILK ALLERGY DIETS;
CHOLESTEROL REDUCTION; HYPERTENSION REDUCTION.

Mushroom Stroganoff (V 4)

Many years ago when I ate meat a good stroganoff was my favourite meal.
Not to lose out I invented this dish which contains none of the 'baddies'
and tastes delicious.

Preparation Time: 15 minutes
Cooking Time: 30 minutes
Ingredients: Imperial/Metric
2oz/50g   polyunsaturated margarine (unhydrogenated)
1   large onion, peeled and sliced
2   garlic cloves, peeled and crushed
1lb/450g   button mushrooms, wiped and sliced
6oz/175g   fresh tomatoes, wiped and sliced
5fl oz/150ml silken tofu, liquidized
1tbsp   fresh chives, chopped
              black pepper and low sodium salt

Method

1 Heat the margarine and add the onion and garlic. Fry gently for 5
  minutes.
2 Add the mushrooms and cook for 3 minutes.
3 Add the tomatoes and cook gently for 5 minutes.
4 Stir in the tofu and chives and gently heat through, but do not allow to
  boil.
5 Season to taste and serve hot with brown rice.

NUTRITION BOX (per serving)

	Quantity	% RDA		Quantity	% RDA
Calories	152	6.1	Copper	0.81mcg	40.4
Protein	4.8g	7.7	Zinc	0.3mcg	2.9
Total fat	12.1g	16.2	Vitamin A	156.3mg	20.8
made up of:			Vitamin C	8.8mg	29.4
saturated	2.9g	–	Vitamin D	1.0mcg	9.9
polyunsat.	6.5g	–	Vitamin E	11.9mg	98.9
mono-unsat.	2.5g	–	Vitamin B$_1$	0.20mg	20.2
Cholesterol	–	–	Vitamin B$_2$	0.50mg	34.8
Fibre	4.3g	14.4	Nicotinic acid	34.9mg	34.9
Iron	1.9mg	18.4	Vitamin B$_6$	0.22mg	10.8
Calcium	40.4mg	8.1	Vitamin B$_{12}$	0.62mcg	31.2
Magnesium	32.9mg	10.9	Folic acid	38.4mg	12.8
Potassium	772.0mg	25.7	Starch	1.0g	–
Sodium	117.7mg	9.8	Sugars	4.1g	–

USEFUL FOR: HYPERTENSION REDUCTION; CHOLESTEROL REDUCTION; CANCER PREVENTION; HEART DISEASE PREVENTION; STROKE PREVENTION; DAIRY FOOD ALLERGY DIETS; COELIACS.

TIP BOX

Bruise or crush the garlic clove to obtain the strongest flavour.

Stuffed Savoy (F V 4)

Impressive parcels filled with layers of different flavours and textures.

Preparation Time: 35 minutes
Cooking Time: 60 minutes
Temperature: 180°C, 350°F, Gas Mark 4
Ingredients: Imperial/Metric

4	outer leaves from a Savoy cabbage, washed
1	large carrot, washed
2tbsp	extra virgin olive oil
1tbsp	onion, peeled and finely sliced
3tbsp	wholemeal breadcrumbs
2tbsp	sunflower seeds, roasted
1tsp	tamari (strong soy sauce)
½	lemon (well scrubbed) zest and juice
3tbsp	silken tofu, liquidized
1tbsp	wholemeal flour
4oz/125g	mushrooms, wiped and finely chopped
1tsp	freshly grated nutmeg
	black pepper and low sodium salt

Method

1 Plunge cabbage leaves in boiling water for 5 minutes then place under cold running water to fix colour. Carefully cut out the central stalks.
2 Cut the carrot into matchstick lengths, about ¼in thick. Cook in boiling water for about 10 minutes. Drain and reserve liquid for stock.
3 Heat the oil, add the onion, and fry gently for 5 minutes.
4 Mix together onions, breadcrumbs, seeds, tamari, lemon rind and juice.
5 Place tofu in a small saucepan. Heat through and add the flour, stirring, until the sauce thickens. Add the mushrooms and cook for 3 minutes.
6 Remove from heat and add the nutmeg and seasoning. Leave to cool.
7 Spread the cabbage leaves out flat. Divide the breadcrumb mixture between them, placing the mixture in the centre of each loaf. Press down very firmly.
8 Arrange a layer of carrot on the top.
9 Finish with a layer of tofu. Carefully fold up the cabbage tightly, like a parcel.
10 Cook in a shallow ovenproof dish, with a little hot water in the base, for 30 minutes. Serve with fresh vegetables and some garlic and tofu dip (p. 48) to which you have added a good squeeze of lemon juice.

NUTRITION BOX (per serving)					
	Quantity	% RDA		Quantity	% RDA
Calories	150	6.0	Copper	0.37mcg	18.4
Protein	3.6g	5.7	Zinc	0.61mcg	6.1
Total fat	8.3g	11.1	Vitamin A	1250.7mg	166.6
made up of:			Vitamin C	51.1mg	170.2
saturated	1.2g	–	Vitamin D	–	–
polyunsat.	1.3g	–	Vitamin E	6.4mg	53.7
mono-unsat.	5.6	–	Vitamin B_1	0.28mg	28.3
Cholesterol	–	–	Vitamin B_2	0.19mg	13.6
Fibre	5.3g	17.8	Nicotinic Acid	2.2mg	13.4
Iron	2.0mg	19.2	Vitamin B_6	0.18mg	9.1
Calcium	82.5mg	16.5	Vitamin B_{12}	–	–
Magnesium	34.2mg	11.4	Folic acid	34.2mg	11.4
Potassium	401.3mg	13.4	Starch	6.8g	–
Sodium	88.8mg	7.4	Sugars	17.1g	–

USEFUL FOR: CANCER PREVENTION; HEART DISEASE PREVENTION; STROKE PREVENTION; DAIRY FOOD ALLERGY DIETS; CHOLESTEROL REDUCTION; HYPERTENSION REDUCTION.

TIP BOX

Increase your fibre intake gradually over some weeks rather than suddenly. This way you will avoid initial digestive problems.

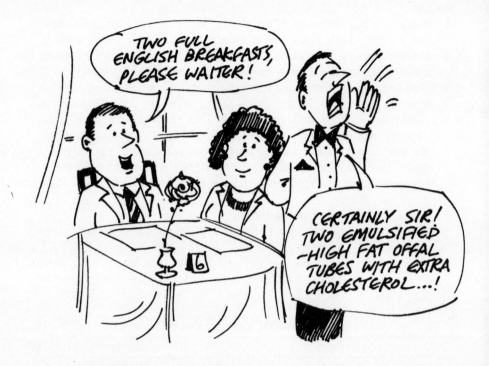

Tomato and Carrot Flan (F V 4)

A very colourful flan with lots of taste and a variety of textures.

Preparation Time: 40 minutes
Cooking Time: 30 minutes
Temperature: 200°C, 400°F, Gas Mark 6
Setting Time: 60 minutes
Ingredients: Imperial/Metric

1 quantity	low fat pastry
1tbsp	extra virgin olive oil
3oz/75g	onion, peeled and chopped
2	garlic cloves, peeled and crushed
8oz/225g	tomatoes, washed and chopped
4oz/100g	carrots, washed and grated
4oz/100g	red lentils, washed and cooked
1tbsp	tomato purée
	black pepper
½pt/250ml	water
1tbsp	fresh mint, washed and chopped
1tbsp	Gelozone

Method

1 Roll out the pastry and line a 20cm (8in) flan dish. Prick the base.
2 Bake in the hottest part of a preheated oven for 20 minutes. (Even in fan-assisted ovens the top is usually the hottest part. It is important for the sides of the flan to cook, otherwise they will collapse.) Leave to cool.
3 Heat the oil in a medium-sized saucepan. Fry the onion and garlic for 5 minutes.
4 Add the tomatoes, carrots, lentils, tomato purée and water. Bring to the boil and gently simmer.
5 Add the mint and stir in the Gelozone very quickly with a fork to ensure it dissolves completely. Simmer for 3 minutes.
6 Pour the mixture into the pastry case and leave for about 1 hour to set.

NUTRITION BOX (per serving)					
	Quantity	% RDA		Quantity	% RDA
Calories	131	5.2	Copper	0.2mcg	11.8
Protein	6.9g	11.1	Zinc	1.0mcg	10.2
Total fat	4.0g	5.3	Vitamin A	558.7mg	74.5
made up of:			Vitamin C	3.1mg	10.2
saturated	0.5g	–	Vitamin D	–	–
polyunsat.	0.4g	–	Vitamin E	11.6mg	96.4
mono-unsat.	2.8g	–	Vitamin B$_1$	0.2mg	18.6
Cholesterol	–	–	Vitamin B$_2$	0.1mg	6.5
Fibre	4.8g	16.0	Nicotinic acid	2.1mg	12.8
Iron	22.7mg	22.7	Vitamin B$_6$	0.3mg	12.7
Calcium	32.9mg	6.6	Vitamin B$_{12}$	–	–
Magnesium	28.7mg	9.6	Folic Acid	26.8mg	8.9
Potassium	392.6mg	13.1	Starch	13.7g	–
Sodium	25.7mg	2.1	Sugars	4.2g	–
USEFUL FOR: CANCER PREVENTION; MILK ALLERGY DIETS; HYPERTENSION REDUCTION.					

Vegetable Lasagne (F 8)

Everybody seems to love a lasagne. This particular one is very colourful with the reds and greens of the peppers contrasting with the creamy white sauce.

Preparation Time: 45 minutes
Cooking Time: 40 minutes
Temperature: 190°C, 375°F, Gas Mark 5
Ingredients: Imperial/Metric
8oz/225g   carrots, washed and diced
8oz/225g   courgettes, washed and sliced
1   onion, peeled and chopped
3   garlic cloves, peeled and crushed
1   red pepper, washed, deseeded and sliced

1	green pepper, washed, deseeded and sliced
5fl oz/150ml	vegetable stock
1oz/25g	polyunsaturated margarine (unhydrogenated)
2tbsp	wholemeal flour
10fl oz/250ml	soya milk (sugar free)
2tsp	dried thyme
2tsp	dried chives
6 oz/175g	wholewheat lasagne
3oz/75g	low fat vegetarian cheese, grated
3oz/75g	low fat vegetarian soft cheese
	black pepper and low sodium salt

Method

1 Place the vegetables in a saucepan with the stock. Bring to the boil and simmer for 10 minutes, covered.

2 Melt the margarine in a pan and add the flour. Cook for 1 minute, stirring all the time. Remove from the heat.

3 Gradually stir in the milk. Return to the heat, bring to the boil and simmer for about 5 minutes, until the sauce thickens, stirring frequently. Season and add the herbs.

4 Cook the lasagne as directed on the packet. Drain.

5 In a large, shallow, ovenproof dish make alternative layers of vegetables, lasagne and cheese – finishing with a layer of lasagne.

6 Pour on the sauce and cook until piping hot and bubbling – about 40 minutes.

7 Serve with a crisp mixed salad.

NUTRITION BOX (per serving)					
	Quantity	% RDA		Quantity	% RDA
Calories	152	6.1	Copper	0.11mcg	5.7
Protein	7.9g	12.6	Zinc	0.6mcg	5.8
Total fat	4.4g	4.4	Vitamin A	1240.4mg	165.4
made up of:			Vitamin C	42.4mg	141.5
saturated	0.4g	–	Vitamin D	0.1mcg	1.6
polyunsat.	1.2g	–	Vitamin E	0.9mg	7.7
mono-unsat.	0.4g	–	Vitamin B_1	0.18mg	18.4
Cholesterol	–	–	Vitamin B_2	0.21mg	14.3
Fibre	6.6g	22.2	Nicotinic Acid	1.8mg	10.9
Iron	4.5mg	43.3	Vitamin B_6	0.26mg	13.1
Calcium	143.0mg	28.6	Vitamin B_{12}	0.2mcg	9.1
Magnesium	27.1mg	9.0	Folic Acid	68.4mg	22.8
Potassium	449.9mg	15.0	Starch	10.1g	–
Sodium	114.2mg	9.5	Sugars	18.3g	–
USEFUL FOR: CHOLESTEROL REDUCTION; HYPERTENSION REDUCTION; CANCER PREVENTION; HEART DISEASE PREVENTION; STROKE PREVENTION.					

Spiced Vegetable Bake (F 4)

This dish, a subtle blend of spices and vegetables with a slightly tart topping, was invented on a wing and a prayer – literally! Unexpected guests, requiring an evening meal, arrived and I had to conjure up something for them fast. It's now a regular on the menu at Harrow Ings.

Preparation Time: 40 minutes
Cooking time: 40 minutes
Temperature: 200°C, 400°F, Gas Mark 6
Ingredients: Imperial/Metric

1	aubergine
3tbsp	extra virgin olive oil (2tbsp for frying, 1tbsp for the aubergines)
2tsp	cumin seeds
2tsp	maram gasala
2	onions, peeled and sliced
3	garlic cloves, peeled and crushed
12oz/350g	pumpkin, peeled, deseeded and diced or swede, peeled and diced
2tbsp	raisins
3tbsp	fresh parsley, chopped
	black pepper
8oz/225g	fromage frais (1% fat variety)

Method:

1 Wipe and slice the aubergine into rounds of about 6mm (¼in) thickness. Brush a baking tray with oil and place the aubergine slices onto it. Brush with oil. Cook in a preheated oven for about 30 minutes. Leave to one side.
2 Heat the remaining oil in a large saucepan. Add the cumin seeds and maram gasala and cook for 3 minutes.
3 Add the onion and garlic and fry gently for 5 minutes.
4 Add the pumpkin (or swede). Stir well and cook, covered, for about 30 minutes – until the pumpkin is just tender.
5 Add the raisins and cook gently for 10 minutes.
6 Remove from the heat and stir in the chopped parsley and seasoning.
7 Divide the pumpkin mixture between four individual ovenproof dishes. Place a layer of aubergine on the top of each.
8 Spoon the fromage frais over the mixture.
9 Place in the oven and cook until the topping is golden brown and just beginning to crisp up.
10 Serve hot together with a baked potato and parsnips sprinkled with lemon juice.

NUTRITION BOX (per serving)					
	Quantity	% RDA		Quantity	% RDA
Calories	251	10.0	Copper	0.23mcg	11.6
Protein	6.5g	10.4	Zinc	0.37mcg	3.7
Total fat	11.8g	15.7	Vitamin A	278.0mg	37.1
made up of:			Vitamin C	25.2mg	83.9
saturated	1.6g	–	Vitamin D	–	–
polyunsat.	1.2g	–	Vitamin E	0.69mg	5.8
mono-unsat.	8.4g	–	Vitamin B_1	0.12mg	12.6
Cholesterol	–	–	Vitamin B_2	0.11mg	8.1
Fibre	4.2g	14.1	Nicotinic Acid	1.5mg	9.4
Iron	1.6mg	16.0	Vitamin B_6	0.20mg	10.3
Calcium	89.7mg	17.9	Vitamin B_{12}	–	–
Magnesium	26.7mg	8.9	Folic Acid	27.2mg	9.1
Potassium	703.5mg	23.4	Starch	4.5g	–
Sodium	16.5mg	1.4	Sugars	12.3g	–

USEFUL FOR: CANCER PREVENTION; COELIACS; HYPERTENSION
REDUCTION; CHOLESTEROL REDUCTION.

TIP BOX

Garlic has been known for its healing powers for centuries in many cultures. Garlic reduces the LDL type of cholesterol, the 'bad' one, and increases the 'good' type, HDL, and is also beneficial in treating heart disease. It is also well known for its antibiotic qualities.

Vegetable Crumble (F V 4)

The crunchy topping has a nutty taste and the garlic gives it a nice 'bite'. The vegetables taste better if they are slightly undercooked.

Preparation Time: 25 minutes
Cooking Time: 30 minutes
Temperature: 180°C, 350°F, Gas Mark 4
Ingredients: Imperial/Metric
2oz/50g	polyunsaturated margarine (unhydrogenated)
1	large onion
1	red pepper
1	green pepper
6oz/175g	button mushrooms, wiped
6oz/175g	fresh tomatoes
	black pepper and low sodium salt

Topping

6oz/175g	wholemeal breadcrumbs
2	garlic cloves, peeled and crushed
4oz/125g	mixed seeds (pumpkin, sunflower, for example), ground

Method

1. Wash and dice all the vegetables.
2. Melt the margarine in a saucepan and fry the onion and peppers for 3 minutes, gently.
3. Add the mushrooms and seasoning. Cook for 3 minutes.
4. Add the tomatoes and cook for 5 minutes, stirring gently.
5. Place the mixture into four individual ovenproof dishes.
6. Mix together all the topping ingredients and divide it between the four dishes.
7. Cook in a preheated oven until heated through and golden brown on the top.
8. Serve with jacket potatoes and a selection of lightly steamed vegetables.

NUTRITION BOX (per serving)					
	Quantity	% RDA		Quantity	% RDA
Calories	310	12.4	Copper	26.3mcg	26.3
Protein	6.2g	9.9	Zinc	1.2mcg	12.1
Total fat	12.2g	16.2	Vitamin A	206.9mg	27.6
made up of:			Vitamin C	238.1mg	238.1
saturated	2.9g	–	Vitamin D	1.0mcg	9.9
polyunsat.	6.1g	–	Vitamin E	22.1mg	184.2
mono-unsat.	2.5g	–	Vitamin B_1	0.82mg	82.2
Cholesterol	–	–	Vitamin B_2	0.34mg	23.3
Fibre	5.5g	18.3	Nicotinic Acid	3.8mg	23.3
Iron	4.4mg	42.5	Vitamin B_6	0.30mg	15.2
Calcium	78.3mg	15.6	Vitamin B_{12}	0.62mcg	31.2
Magnesium	24.7mg	24.7	Folic Acid	45.9mg	15.3
Potassium	927.1mg	30.9	Starch	18.4g	–
Sodium	348.9mg	29.1	Sugars	6.3g	–

USEFUL FOR: CANCER PREVENTION; HEART DISEASE PREVENTION; STROKE PREVENTION; DAIRY FOOD ALLERGY DIETS; CHOLESTEROL REDUCTION; HYPERTENSION REDUCTION.

TIP BOX

In spite of its name, buckwheat flour does not contain wheat and can be used by coeliacs.

Basic Buckwheat Pancake Mixture (F V 4)

Pancakes are wonderful because they are versatile, as well as quick and easy to make. Try using different fillings and sauces – the combinations are endless. Buckwheat flour gives the pancakes a 'nutty' flavour which I find delicious, but you can use other flours and each will give a subtly different taste.

Preparation Time: 10 minutes
Cooking Time: 10 minutes
Ingredients: Imperial/Metric
4oz/125g   buckwheat flour
½pt/250ml   soya milk (sugar free)
2tsp   extra virgin olive oil
                  little oil for frying
                  black pepper

Method

1 Sift the flour into a bowl.
2 Gradually add the milk and beat well until the mixture is smooth.
3 Add the black pepper and oil.
4 Continue to whisk the mixture to let more air into the batter.
5 Melt a little oil in a non-stick frying pan and pour in a thin layer of the batter. Cook gently on one side, and when cooked toss, or turn with a wooden spatula, and cook the other side.
6 Keep the pancakes warm while you make the remainder. A good way to do this is to turn the grill on high before you start making the pancakes. Then, just before the first one is cooked, turn the grill low and slip the pancakes onto a plate under the grill as you make them.

NUTRITION BOX (per serving)					
	Quantity	% RDA		Quantity	% RDA
Calories	182	7.3	Copper	0.2mcg	8.8
Protein	8.0g	12.7	Zinc	1.3mcg	13.3
Total fat	4.6g	6.2	Vitamin A	–	–
made up of:			Vitamin C	–	–
saturated	0.5g	–	Vitamin D	–	–
polyunsat.	1.8g	–	Vitamin E	0.6mg	4.7
mono-unsat.	1.9g	–	Vitamin B$_1$	0.2mg	22.6
Cholesterol	–	–	Vitamin B$_2$	0.04mg	3.3
Fibre	3.9g	13.0	Nicotinic Acid	1.1mg	6.6
Iron	2.4mg	23.0	Vitamin B$_6$	0.6mg	29.7
Calcium	61.2mg	12.3	Vitamin B$_{12}$	–	–
Magnesium	73.1mg	24.4	Folic Acid	24.9mg	8.3
Potassium	174.1mg	5.8	Starch	27.8g	–
Sodium	4.5mg	0.4	Sugars	157.5g	–
USEFUL FOR: DAIRY FOOD ALLERGY DIETS; HYPERTENSION REDUCTION.					

Broccoli and Mushroom Pancake Filling (F 4)
Just one of the many possible pancake fillings to give you inspiration!

Preparation Time: 15 minutes
Cooking Time: 25 minutes
Temperature: 150°C, 300°C, Gas Mark 2
Ingredients: Imperial/Metric

4oz/100g	broccoli, washed and cut into small florets.
8oz/225g	mushrooms, wiped and sliced
3oz/75g	sunflower seeds, roasted
8oz/225g	fromage frais (1% fat variety)
2oz/50g	low fat vegetarian cheese, grated
	black pepper

Method
1 Steam the broccoli for about 5 minutes.
2 Make the pancakes as in the recipe on p. 00.
3 Mix together the mushrooms, broccoli, seeds, cheeses and black pepper.
4 Place a spoonful of the mixture onto half of each pancake.
5 Fold the pancake to cover the mixture.
6 Place the pancakes in a shallow ovenproof dish and cook for about 20 minutes until heated through.

NUTRITION BOX (per serving)					
	Quantity	% RDA		Quantity	% RDA
Calories	118	4.7	Copper	0.4mcg	19.2
Protein	9.7g	15.5	Zinc	0.7mcg	6.6
Total fat	2.8g	3.7	Vitamin A	187.1mg	24.9
made up of:			Vitamin C	12.9mg	43.1
saturated	0.1g	–	Vitamin D	0.02mcg	.2
polyunsat.	0.2g	–	Vitamin E	6.2mg	51.6
mono-unsat.	–	–	Vitamin B_1	0.4mg	44.4
Cholesterol	–	–	Vitamin B_2	0.4mg	25.4
Fibre	2.4g	8.1	Nicotinic Acid	3.6mg	22.0
Iron	2.2mg	20.9	Vitamin B_6	0.1mg	5.1
Calcium	135.7mg	27.1	Vitamin B_{12}	0.2mcg	8.8
Magnesium	20.9mg	7.0	Folic Acid	42.9mg	14.3
Potassium	511.9mg	17.1	Starch	1.8g	–
Sodium	129.1mg	10.8	Sugars	0.4g	–
USEFUL FOR: CANCER PREVENTION; HEART DISEASE PREVENTION; STROKE PREVENTION; COELIACS; CHOLESTEROL REDUCTION; HYPERTENSION REDUCTION.					

Butter Bean Rissoles (F V 4)

A delicate mixture of pale greens and pale yellows, these rissoles are crisp on the outside and beautifully soft on the inside.

Preparation time: 20 minutes
Cooking Time: 8 minutes
Ingredients Imperial/Metric

8oz/225g	butter beans, soaked and cooked – reserve the liquid
1tbsp	tahini
3tbsp	fresh parsley, chopped
3	garlic cloves, peeled and crushed
1tsp	dried basil
1tsp	saffron
1tbsp	soya milk (sugar free)
1tbsp	sesame seeds or millet flakes
1tbsp	extra virgin olive oil

Method

1 Mash the butter beans with 4 tbsp of the reserved cooking liquid.
2 Add the tahini, parsley, garlic, basil and saffron. Mix well.
3 Form into 8 rissole (burger) shapes.
4 Brush with the soya milk and coat with the seeds or flakes.
5 Shallow fry in the oil for 4 minutes on each side.
6 Serve hot with either a salad or vegetables.

NUTRITION BOX (per serving)					
	Quantity	% RDA		Quantity	% RDA
Calories	229	9.2	Copper	0.71mcg	35.3
Protein	11.2g	17.9	Zinc	1.6mcg	16.4
Total fat	4.4g	5.9	Vitamin A	41.2mg	5.5
made up of:			Vitamin C	6.0mg	20.0
saturated	0.5g	–	Vitamin D	–	–
polyunsat.	0.5g	–	Vitamin E	1.4mg	11.8
mono-unsat.	2.8g	–	Vitamin B_1	0.34mg	34.3
Cholesterol	–	–	Vitamin B_2	0.1mg	6.6
Fibre	12.5g	41.6	Nicotinic Acid	3.2mg	19.6
Iron	4.0mg	38.6	Vitamin B_6	0.35mg	17.8
Calcium	68.1mg	13.6	Vitamin B_{12}	–	–
Magnesium	96.6mg	32.2	Folic Acid	62.1mg	20.7
Potassium	1046.2mg	34.9	Starch	27.0g	–
Sodium	37.0mg	3.1	Sugars	2.0g	–

USEFUL FOR: HEART DISEASE PREVENTION; COELIACS; DAIRY FOOD ALLERGY DIETS; HYPERTENSION REDUCTION; CHOLESTEROL REDUCTION.

Tomato and Seed Rissoles (F 4)

These rissoles are also good sandwiched inside a wholemeal bap with some onions and relish.

Preparation Time: 15 minutes
Cooking Time: 10 minutes
Ingredients: Imperial/Metric

4oz/125g	sunflower seeds, ground
2oz/50g	vegetarian low fat cheese
2oz/50g	vegetarian low fat soft cheese
4	tomatoes, chopped
2	garlic cloves, peeled and crushed
1tbsp	tomato purée (sugar free)
1oz/25g	onion, grated
2tsp	mixed herbs
1tbsp	tahini
3oz/75g	wholemeal breadcrumbs
1tbsp	soya milk (sugar free)
2tbsp	olive oil for frying
1	lemon (well scrubbed) zest and juice
	black pepper

Method

1 Mix all the ingredients, except for 1oz (25g) of the breadcrumbs, together in a bowl.
2 Form into eight evenly sized 'burger' shapes.
3 Brush each with a little soya milk and coat with the remaining breadcrumbs.
4 Shallow fry until they are crisp and golden brown.
5 Serve hot garnished with slices of tomato.

NUTRITION BOX (per serving)					
	Quantity	% RDA		Quantity	% RDA
Calories	272	10.9	Copper	0.12mcg	6.2
Protein	7.9g	12.6	Zinc	1.0mcg	10.3
Total fat	9.8g	13.1	Vitamin A	85.9mg	11.4
made up of:			Vitamin C	3.9mg	13.1
saturated	0.7g	–	Vitamin D	0.02mcg	0.22
polyunsat.	1.0g	–	Vitamin E	21.4mg	178.2
mono-unsat.	4.7g	–	Vitamin B_1	0.71mg	71.5
Cholesterol	–	–	Vitamin B_2	0.16mg	11.2
Fibre	10.9g	10.9	Nicotinic Acid	1.5mg	9.4
Iron	3.0mg	29.6	Vitamin B_6	0.14mg	7.0
Calcium	152.0mg	30.4	Vitamin B_{12}	0.17mcg	8.7
Magnesium	41.2mg	13.7	Folic Acid	25.8mg	8.6
Potassium	544.4mg	18.1	Starch	9.0g	–
Sodium	227.3mg	18.9	Sugars	2.4g	–
USEFUL FOR: HEART DISEASE PREVENTION; HYPERTENSION REDUCTION.					

7
NAKED VEGETABLES

All too often the vegetables accompanying a main meal are not given a second thought. Rather than being there just to fill the plate up they should actually complement the main dish and supply various nutrients.

Fresh vegetables in season are wonderful and take very little preparation and cooking. Most fresh vegetables can be cooked as quickly as tinned vegetables. The advantage of using fresh is that you retain important vitamins, minerals and fibre, without the problem of added sugar, salt and preservatives. The taste is totally different as well. Fresh vegetables are tasty, crisp and appetizing, and tend to be cheaper than their tinned counterparts.

There are many interesting vegetables on the market these days from all over the world and they are certainly worth trying. Experiment with them - be adventurous for it is well worth the effort.

Common problems

The most common problem when it comes to vegetables is overcooking. The only thing that is worse than looking at a plate of limp, lifeless vegetables is eating them. Vegetables should be fresh looking, crisp and colourful. The secret is to cook them for the shortest time possible. This not only retains their flavour but also their nutrients.

The best way to cook vegetables is by steaming them briefly over a pan of boiling water. They should be steamed until just tender but retaining their crispness. Keep testing vegetables by piercing them with a sharp pointed knife. Vegetables which are boiled lose a lot of their nutrients in the cooking liquid and have a tendency to be limp.

When preparing vegetables cut away as little as possible. Most vegetables need only washing or at the most scraping. When slicing vegetables like carrots or courgettes cut them lengthways rather than in circles. They not only cook more quickly but they also retain more of their nutrients.

From the way vegetables so often get plonked on a plate, you'd think their presentation was a problem, but it really isn't. When you are planning a meal think of the colours that will be together on the plate. Will they complement each other? Will the plate look too dull? Personally, I like to see contrasting colours such as the dark green of spring cabbage with the vibrant orange of carrots. I would never serve cauliflower, sweetcorn and mashed potato on the same plate - the colours are much too similar.

Once you have thought about the colours then you have to arrange them attractively on the plate, not only bearing in mind colour but also textures

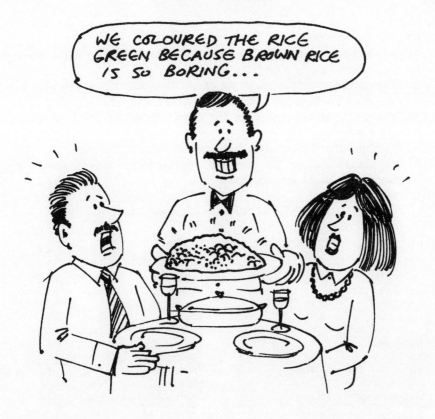

and shapes. Serve chopped root vegetables with leafy vegetables. And if one of the vegetables is served with a sauce the others should be served 'au naturel'. It is easy to 'overdo' the use of sauces. There is nothing wrong with 'naked' vegetables – they taste delicious.

Aubergine with Tomatoes (F V 8)
Aubergine and tomatoes provide a colourful accompaniment to any main course. In fact, served with garlic bread, this dish is substantial enough for a main course.

Preparation Time: 20 minutes
Cooking Time: 25 minutes
Temperature: 230°C, 460°F, Gas Mark 8
Ingredients: Imperial/Metric

2	aubergines, washed
8oz/225g	tomatoes, washed and halved
ltbsp/15ml	sesame seed oil
2tsp	dried basil
	black pepper and low sodium salt

87

Method

1 Slice the aubergines into rings 6mm (¼in) thick.
2 Cut the tomatoes in half.
3 Brush three baking trays with oil.
4 Arrange the aubergine slices on two of the baking trays, making sure that you do not overlap them. Brush lightly with oil.
5 Arrange the tomato halves on the remaining baking tray and sprinkle with the basil.
6 Place in the preheated oven and cook for 15 minutes.
7 Mix the aubergines and tomatoes together with the seasonings and arrange in a warm serving dish.

NUTRITION BOX (per serving)					
	Quantity	% RDA		Quantity	% RDA
Calories	70.6	2.8	Copper	0.1mcg	4.4
Protein	0.8g	1.2	Zinc	0.1mcg	0.6
Total fat	6.2g	8.3	Vitamin A	28.1mg	3.8
made up of:			Vitamin C	3.8mg	12.5
saturated	0.9g	–	Vitamin D	–	–
polyunsat.	0.7g	–	Vitamin E	5.9mg	49.5
mono-unsat.	4.7g	–	Vitamin B_1	0.1mg	5.4
Cholesterol	–	–	Vitamin B_2	0.03mg	2.3
Fibre	2.3g	7.7	Nicotinic Acid	0.9mg	5.5
Iron	0.4mg	4.0	Vitamin B_6	0.1mg	4.5
Calcium	11.2mg	2.2	Vitamin B_{12}	–	–
Magnesium	10.6mg	3.5	Folic Acid	22.9mg	7.6
Potassium	261.6mg	8.7	Starch	0.2g	–
Sodium	3.1mg	0.3	Sugars	3.0g	–
USEFUL FOR: COELIACS; DAIRY FOOD ALLERGY DIETS.					

Broccoli with Mint and Yogurt (4)

Yogurt and fresh mint go very well together and make an interesting dressing for salads and vegetables alike.

Preparation Time: 20 minutes
Cooking Time: 15 minutes
Ingredients: Imperial/Metric
1lb/500g   broccoli, well washed
5fl oz/150ml natural, unsweetened low fat yogurt
1tbsp   fresh mint, chopped
           black pepper
1   sprig fresh mint

Method

1 Place the broccoli in a steamer and steam over a pan of boiling water for 15 minutes.

2 Gently heat the yogurt in a small saucepan. Add the mint and pepper.
3 Place the broccoli in a warm serving dish and pour over the mint and yogurt sauce.
4 Garnish with a sprig of mint.

NUTRITION BOX (per serving)					
	Quantity	% RDA		Quantity	% RDA
Calories	42	1.7	Copper	0.12mcg	5.8
Protein	5.8g	9.3	Zinc	0.7mcg	7.3
Total fat	0.4g	.5	Vitamin A	790.9mg	103.5
made up of:			Vitamin C	56.4mg	188.0
saturated	–	–	Vitamin D	–	–
polyunsat.	–	–	Vitamin E	1.4mg	11.6
mono-unsat.	–	–	Vitamin B	0.1mg	8.3
Cholesterol	–	–	Vitamin B$_2$	0.3mg	24.0
Fibre	5.1g	17.1	Nicotinic Acid	1.9mg	11.7
Iron	1.3mg	12.5	Vitamin B$_6$	0.2mg	8.9
Calcium	162.5mg	32.5	Vitamin B$_{12}$	–	–
Magnesium	21.4mg	7.1	Folic Acid	138.3mg	46.1
Potassium	365.0mg	12.2	Starch	0.1g	–
Sodium	36.0mg	3.0	Sugars	1.9g	–

USEFUL FOR: CANCER PREVENTION; HYPERTENSION REDUCTION; COELIACS.

TIP BOX

Vegetables should be used as quickly as possible after being picked, otherwise they lose nutrients.

Carrots with Orange and Ginger (F V 4)

The carrots absorb the orange juice and ginger during cooking which gives them a distinctive flavour. By serving with the cooking juice, you will retain the nutrients lost during cooking.

Preparation Time: 10 minutes
Cooking Time: 20 minutes
Ingredients: Imperial/Metric
1lb/450g   carrots, washed
½pt/250ml   orange juice, unsweetened
2tsp   ground ginger
1tsp   stem ginger, chopped
                black pepper

Method

1 Cut the carrots into fingers about 5cm (2in) long and 6mm (¼in) thick.
2 Place half the carrots in a medium-sized saucepan. Sprinkle with black pepper and half the ground ginger.
3 Place the remaining carrots in the saucepan and sprinkle on the remaining ground ginger and the black pepper.
4 Pour on the orange juice.
5 Bring to the boil and simmer for about 20 minutes, until the carrots are tender but not soft.
6 Place the carrots and the juice in a serving dish and sprinkle the choopped stem ginger on the top.

NUTRITION BOX (per serving)					
	Quantity	% RDA		Quantity	% RDA
Calories	44.4	1.8	Copper	0.1mcg	5.9
Protein	0.1g	1.6	Zinc	0.6mcg	5.6
Total fat	–	–	Vitamin A	334.0mg	334.0
made up of:			Vitamin C	83.3mg	83.3
saturated	–	–	Vitamin D	–	–
polyunsat.	–	–	Vitamin E	5.2mg	5.2
mono-unsat.	–	–	Vitamin B_1	0.1mg	10.6
Cholesterol	–	–	Vitamin B_2	0.1mg	4.3
Fibre	3.9g	12.9	Nicotinic Acid	0.8mg	4.9
Iron	0.8mg	7.9	Vitamin B_6	0.1mg	6.9
Calcium	51.9mg	10.4	Vitamin B_{12}	–	–
Magnesium	13.1mg	4.4	Folic Acid	14.4mg	4.8
Potassium	190.0mg	6.3	Starch	0.1g	–
Sodium	65.0mg	5.4	Sugars	10.6g	–
USEFUL FOR: CANCER PREVENTION; COELIACS; DAIRY FOOD ALLERGY DIETS.					

Cheese and Celery Baked Potato (4)

Baked potatoes lend themselves to a variety of fillings. This one combines the flavours of cheese and onion.

Preparation Time: 20 minutes
Cooking Time: 70 minutes
Temperature: 200°C, 400°F, Gas Mark 6
Ingredients: Imperial/Metric

4	potatoes, large enough to bake, washed
2	celery sticks, washed and grated
4oz/100g	vegetarian low fat soft cheese
2tsp	paprika pepper
1tbsp	fresh chives, chopped

Method

1 Place a skewer through each potato and place in the preheated oven for 1 hour, or until the potatoes are cooked through.
2 Meanwhile mix together the remaining ingredients.
3 Carefully scoop out the potato leaving a 'shell'.
4 Add this potato to the cheese mixture and mix well.
5 Pile this mixture into each of the potato 'shells' and return to the oven for 10 minutes.
6 Sprinkle each with some chopped fresh chives.

NUTRITION BOX (per serving)					
	Quantity	% RDA		Quantity	% RDA
Calories	80.8	3.2	Copper	4.5mcg	4.5
Protein	3.9g	6.2	Zinc	0.1mcg	1.4
Total fat	2.2g	3.0	Vitamin A	–	–
made up of:			Vitamin C	6.8mg	22.7
saturated	–	–	Vitamin D	–	–
polyunsat.	–	–	Vitamin E	0.1mg	0.9
mono-unsat.	–	–	Vitamin B_1	0.1mg	5.3
Cholesterol	–	–	Vitamin B_2	0.02mg	1.7
Fibre	3.2g	10.6	Nicotinic Acid	0.7mg	4.5
Iron	0.3mg	3.1	Vitamin B_6	0.1mg	6.3
Calcium	15.2mg	3.1	Vitamin B_{12}	–	–
Magnesium	3.6mg	3.6	Folic Acid	8.6mg	2.9
Potassium	8.7mg	8.7	Starch	11.5g	–
Sodium	3.1mg	3.1	Sugars	0.5g	–
USEFUL FOR: HYPERTENSION REDUCTION; COELIACS.					

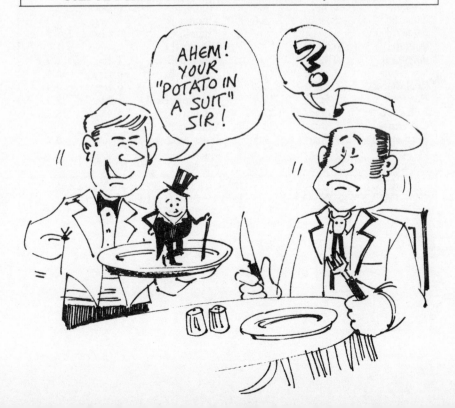

Leeks with Lemon and Raisins (F V 4)

Unusual and tasty, the raisins add a sweetness to the leeks and the lemon adds a nice tang.

Preparation Time: 15 minutes
Cooking Time: 7 minutes
Ingredients: Imperial/Metric

1tbsp	sesame seed oil
1lb/500g	leeks, washed well and chopped
2tsp	caraway seeds
	black pepper
2tbsp	raisins
2	lemons, juice and rind

Method

1 Heat the oil in a wok or large frying pan.
2 Add the leeks and stir fry for 5 minutes.
3 Add the caraway seeds, black pepper and raisins. Stir fry for 2 minutes.
4 Remove from the heat and arrange the leeks in a serving dish.
5 Pour over the lemon juice and sprinkle on the rind. Combine well and serve.

NUTRITION BOX (per serving)					
	Quantity	% RDA		Quantity	% RDA
Calories	205.8	8.2	Copper	0.2mcg	9.7
Protein	2.5g	4.0	Zinc	0.2mcg	1.5
Total fat	3.7g	5.0	Vitamin A	9.4mg	1.3
made up of:		–	Vitamin C	40.8mg	135.8
saturated	0.5g	–	Vitamin D	–	–
polyunsat.	0.4g	–	Vitamin E	1.2mg	9.9
mono-unsat.	2.8g	–	Vitamin B_1	0.1mg	14.5
Cholesterol	–	–	Vitamin B_2	0.1mg	5.4
Fibre	5.5g	18.4	Nicotinic Acid	1.2mg	7.5
Iron	1.6mg	15.9	Vitamin B_6	0.4mg	18.3
Calcium	102.9mg	20.6	Vitamin B_{12}	–	–
Magnesium	19.6mg	6.5	Folic Acid	0.5mg	0.2
Potassium	519.0mg	17.3	Starch	–	–
Sodium	18.7mg	1.6	Sugars	16.0g	–
USEFUL FOR: HYPERTENSION REDUCTION; HEART DISEASE PREVENTION; COELIACS; DAIRY FOOD ALLERGY DIETS.					

Mange-tout and Mushrooms (F V 4)

Also known as snow peas, these are the peas that you eat whole – pod and all – and they cook in no time.

Preparation Time: 5 minutes
Cooking Time: 5 minutes
Ingredients: Imperial/Metric

½tbsp	sesame seed oil, cold pressed
8oz/225g	button mushrooms, wiped
8oz/225g	mange-tout peas, washed
	black pepper

Method

1 Heat the oil in a wok or large frying pan.
2 Add the mushrooms and stir fry for 2 minutes.
3 Add the mange-tout and stir fry for 1 minute.
4 Add the black pepper and stir fry for 1 minute.
5 Arrange in a warm shallow dish and serve.

NUTRITION BOX (per serving)					
	Quantity	% RDA		Quantity	% RDA
Calories	63.5	2.5	Copper	20.8mcg	20.8
Protein	3.8g	6.1	Zinc	0.3mcg	3.4
Total fat	3.5g	4.7	Vitamin A	28.1mg	3.7
made up of:			Vitamin C	9.6mg	31.9
saturated	0.5g	–	Vitamin D	–	–
polyunsat.	0.5g	–	Vitamin E	6.6mg	54.7
mono-unsat.	2.2g	–	Vitamin B_1	0.2mg	19.7
Cholesterol	–	–	Vitamin B_2	6.4mg	442.2
Fibre	4.3g	14.4	Nicotinic Acid	3.9mg	23.5
Iron	1.2mg	12.0	Vitamin B_6	0.1mg	5.6
Calcium	9.0mg	1.8	Vitamin B_{12}	–	–
Magnesium	19.1mg	6.4	Folic Acid	56.8mg	18.9
Potassium	360.0mg	12.0	Starch	1.0g	–
Sodium	5.1mg	0.4	Sugars	1.0g	–

USEFUL FOR: HEART DISEASE PREVENTION; STROKE PREVENTION; CHOLESTEROL REDUCTION; HYPERTENSION REDUCTION; CANCER PREVENTION; COELIACS; DAIRY FOOD ALLERGY DIETS.

Okra and Mushrooms (F V 4)

Okra is sometimes called 'ladies fingers' which aptly describes its shape. When sliced it becomes sticky, so is really nicer whole.

Preparation Time: 10 minutes
Cooking Time: 5 minutes
Ingredients: Imperial/Metric

½tbsp	sesame seed oil
1tsp	cumin seeds
1tsp	maram gasala
8oz/225g	okra, washed and trimmed
8oz/225g	mushrooms, wiped and sliced

Method

1 Heat the oil in a wok or large frying pan.
2 Add the cumin seeds and maram gasala. Fry for 1 minute.
3 Add the okra and stir fry for 2 minutes
4 Add the mushrooms and stir fry for 2 minutes.
5 Arrange in a warm dish and serve.

NUTRITION BOX (per serving)					
	Quantity	% RDA		Quantity	% RDA
Calories	43.8	1.8	Copper	0.5mcg	23.3
Protein	2.1g	3.4	Zinc	0.1mcg	0.6
Total fat	3.3g	4.4	Vitamin A	8.4mg	1.1
made up of:			Vitamin C	15.8mg	52.5
saturated	0.5g	–	Vitamin D	–	–
polyunsat.	0.5g	–	Vitamin E	0.2mg	1.3
mono-unsat.	2.2g	–	Vitamin B$_1$	0.1mg	11.3
Cholesterol	–	–	Vitamin B$_2$	0.3mg	19.4
Fibre	3.2g	10.7	Nicotinic Acid	3.3mg	20.1
Iron	1.1mg	10.9	Vitamin B$_6$	0.1mg	5.1
Calcium	41.1mg	8.2	Vitamin B$_{12}$	–	–
Magnesium	41.1mg	13.7	Folic Acid	69.2mg	23.1
Potassium	371.2mg	12.4	Starch	–	–
Sodium	9.0mg	0.8	Sugars	–	–

USEFUL FOR: CHOLESTEROL REDUCTION; HYPERTENSION REDUCTION; DAIRY FOOD ALLERGY DIETS; COELIACS.

Spinach with Apple (V 4)

An unusual mixture of distinctive flavours which is quick and easy to prepare.

Preparation Time: 6 minutes
Cooking Time: 5 minutes
Ingredients: Imperial/Metric
12oz/350g   spinach, washed and chopped
4oz/100g   red apple, washed, cored and thickly sliced

Method
1 Place the spinach and apple together in a steamer.
2 Steam over a pan of boiling water for 5 minutes.
3 Serve at once.

NUTRITION BOX (per serving)					
	Quantity	% RDA		Quantity	% RDA
Calories	35.5	1.4	Copper	0.3mcg	12.5
Protein	4.5g	7.2	Zinc	0.4mcg	3.8
Total fat	0.4g	0.6	Vitamin A	1051.3mg	140.2
made up of:			Vitamin C	36.1mg	120.4
saturated	0.1g	–	Vitamin D	–	–
polyunsat.	0.3g	–	Vitamin E	1.8mg	14.6
mono-unsat.	–	–	Vitamin B_1	0.1mg	7.1
Cholesterol	–	–	Vitamin B_2	0.1mg	9.4
Fibre	6.2g	20.5	Nicotinic Acid	1.6mg	9.7
Iron	3.6mg	34.7	Vitamin B_6	0.2mg	8.3
Calcium	526.0mg	105.2	Vitamin B_{12}	–	–
Magnesium	52.4mg	17.5	Folic Acid	123.8mg	41.3
Potassium	458.8mg	15.3	Starch	0.2g	–
Sodium	105.5mg	8.9	Sugars	3.5g	–

USEFUL FOR: CANCER PREVENTION; HEART DISEASE PREVENTION; STROKE PREVENTION; HYPERTENSION REDUCTION; CHOLESTEROL REDUCTION; COELIACS; DAIRY FOOD ALLERGY DIETS.

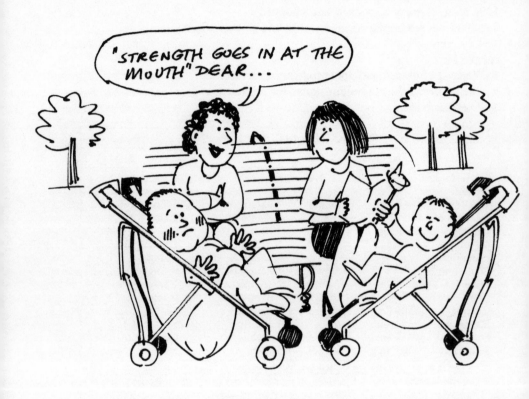

8
SALAD DAYS

Salads are so very versatile that you could have a different one every day of the year. The combination of colours, flavours and textures is endless. Salads can be used as main courses, starters or snacks.

And as for ingredients, you can literally add anything to a salad – beans, lentils, vegetables, fruit, seeds – anything you happen to have in your larder. Use herbs, spices and fruit zests for subtle flavours. The addition of seeds, sprouted beans, raw fruit and raw vegetables will give the salad a crisp and crunchy texture. If you want a smooth, rich, creamy salad then use fromage frais, low fat natural yogurt or tofu as the base and just mix in chopped or puréed fruit and vegetables.

I love making salads. You can really let your artistic streak show and conjure up a work of art. In fact, one of our guests who opted for a vegetarian breakfast exclaimed 'I can't eat this'. I thought, oops what's wrong with it. 'It looks too attractive to eat. Just a minute, I'll go and get my camera.' Yes, he did take a photograph of his breakfast – and did so each morning of his stay with us. After that all the traditional breakfast-eaters wanted the vegetarian breakfast for the remainder of their stay!

Common problems
Too many people think a salad is a piece of lettuce, a slice of tomato, a little cucumber and an onion ring or two, put in a limp pile on your plate. No wonder salad has a bad reputation! Break away from the lettuce and cucumber brigade and experiment with unusual combinations of foods. If you're feeling hesitant, try some of the following recipes, and you'll soon go on to make your own inventions. Presentation really comes to the fore when making salads. You can present a salad beautifully arranged on a single lettuce leaf or nestling in several chicory leaves. You can use a plate to arrange salads using curled spring onions and chicory leaves to give added height and an extra dimension. Well placed 'radish flowers', 'curly celery boats' and 'carrot roses' add a real touch of class – they never fail to impress. And you definitely don't have to spend ages getting the salads ready. I present salads like these as part of my vegetarian breakfasts and they are all made before the meal – if they required hours of presentation I couldn't do it!

Stuffed Apples (4)

A lovely refreshing salad which combines soft cheese, fruits and seeds.

Preparation Time: 15 minutes
Ingredients: Imperial/Metric

4oz/100g	fresh pineapple, peeled and cubed
2	large dessert apples, washed and cored
8oz/225g	low fat soft cheese
3oz/75g	fresh apricots, washed, stoned and chopped
1oz/25g	sunflower seeds
8oz/225g	carrot, washed and grated
2tsp	lemon juice

Method

1 Combine the low fat soft cheese with the pineapple, sunflower seeds and apricots.
2 Cut the apples in half down from the stalk, and carefully scoop out the apple to form four 'shells'. Coat all the apple with the lemon juice.
3 Dice the apple flesh, mix with the soft cheese mixture and pile into the apple shells.
4 Place the grated carrot on a large plate and arrange the stuffed apples on the top. Serve well chilled.

NUTRITION BOX (per serving)					
	Quantity	% RDA		Quantity	% RDA
Calories	139.9	5.6	Copper	0.1mcg	6.7
Protein	7.2g	11.5	Zinc	0.3mcg	2.7
Total fat	4.9g	6.5	Vitamin A	1169.7mg	155.6
made up of:			Vitamin C	7.5mg	25.0
saturated	–	–	Vitamin D	–	–
polyunsat.	–	–	Vitamin E	2.2mg	18.5
mono-unsat.	–	–	Vitamin B_1	0.2mg	19.9
Cholesterol	–	–	Vitamin B_2	0.1mg	4.2
Fibre	8.7g	29.1	Nicotinic Acid	0.5mg	3.0
Iron	1.0mg	9.6	Vitamin B_6	0.1mg	4.9
Calcium	36.4mg	7.3	Vitamin B_{12}	–	–
Magnesium	13.6mg	4.5	Folic Acid	10.4mg	3.5
Potassium	298.3mg	9.9	Starch	1.4g	–
Sodium	29.9mg	2.5	Sugars	11.7g	–
USEFUL FOR: HYPERTENSION REDUCTION; COELIACS.					

Courgette and Melon Salad (V 4)

The tofu gives the salad a nice, light creamy texture without overpowering the taste of the fruits and vegetables.

Preparation Time: 10 minutes
Ingredients: Imperial/Metric

8fl oz/225ml	silken tofu, liquidized
8oz/225g	courgettes, washed and grated
8oz/225g	melon, peeled and chopped
1oz/ 25g	dried prunes, washed, pitted and stoned
1oz/25g	dried dates, washed, pitted and chopped
1 tsp	honey (optional)
4oz/100g	chicory, washed

Method

1 Mix all the ingredients, except the chicory, together.
2 Pile the mixture onto a serving dish and arrange the chicory in it. The mixture will enable you to stand the chicory upright – just stick it in. Arrange some chicory around the edge of the dish.

NUTRITION BOX (per serving)					
	Quantity	% RDA		Quantity	% RDA
Calories	81.6	3.3	Copper	0.1mcg	3.8
Protein	4.3g	6.9	Zinc	0.1mcg	1.3
Total fat	1.7g	2.3	Vitamin A	18.2mg	2.4
made up of:			Vitamin C	24.1mg	80.2
saturated	0.2g	–	Vitamin D	–	–
polyunsat.	1.2g	–	Vitamin E	0.1mg	0.5
mono-unsat.	–	–	Vitamin B_1	0.2mg	19.2
Cholesterol	–	–	Vitamin B_2	0.1mg	5.7
Fibre	2.7g	9.1	Nicotinic Acid	0.1mg	5.1
Iron	2.3mg	22.7	Vitamin B_6	0.1mg	3.1
Calcium	53.9mg	10.8	Vitamin B_{12}	58.2mcg	2909.4
Magnesium	31.4mg	10.5	Folic Acid	58.2mg	19.4
Potassium	392.8mg	13.1	Starch	–	–
Sodium	18.2mg	1.5	Sugars	11.6g	–
USEFUL FOR: HYPERTENSION REDUCTION; COELIACS; DAIRY FOOD ALLERGY DIETS.					

Creamy Vegetable Salad (4)

Fromage frais tastes so rich and creamy that it's hard to believe it contains less than 1% fat.

Preparation Time: 15 minutes
Ingredients: Imperial/Metric

8oz/225g	fromage frais, less than 1% fat variety
4oz/100g	celery, washed and chopped
2oz/50g	chick peas, soaked and cooked
2oz/50g	red lentils, washed and cooked
2oz/50g	parsnips, peeled and grated
4oz/100g	red peppers, washed and chopped
	parsley sprigs or watercress to garnish

Method

1 Mix all the ingredients together, put in a bowl or on a serving dish and garnish with some fresh parsley or watercress.

NUTRITION BOX (per serving)					
	Quantity	% RDA		Quantity	% RDA
Calories	114.9	4.6	Copper	0.2mcg	11.2
Protein	10.3g	16.5	Zinc	0.5mcg	4.8
Total fat	1.5g	2.0	Vitamin A	27.5mg	3.7
made up of:			Vitamin C	32.1mg	107.1
saturated	–	–	Vitamin D	–	–
polyunsat.	–	–	Vitamin E	0.4mg	3.1
mono-unsat.	–	–	Vitamin B_1	0.1mg	14.1
Cholesterol	–	–	Vitamin B_2	0.1mg	4.6
Fibre	4.3g	14.4	Nicotinic Acid	1.7mg	10.4
Iron	2.1mg	20.0	Vitamin B_6	0.2mg	7.5
Calcium	42.1mg	8.4	Vitamin B_{12}	–	–
Magnesium	36.5mg	12.2	Folic Acid	26.4mg	8.8
Potassium	342.5mg	11.4	Starch	14.5g	–
Sodium	45.5mg	3.8	Sugars	2.7g	–
USEFUL FOR: HYPERTENSION REDUCTION; COELIACS.					

Crunchy Salad (V 4)

If you like crunchy salads you will enjoy this one – it is wonderfully refreshing.

Preparation time: 15 minutes
Ingredients: Imperial/Metric

8oz/225g	courgettes, washed and grated
1	red apple, washed, cored and sliced
2	celery sticks, washed and chopped
1	green pepper, washed, deseeded and chopped
2tbsp	pumpkin seeds
2tbsp	sunflower seeds
1	lemon, zest and juice

Method
1 Mix all the ingredients together well and serve in a large shallow dish.

NUTRITION BOX (per serving)					
	Quantity	% RDA		Quantity	% RDA
Calories	71.4	2.9	Copper	0.1mcg	1.8
Protein	1.5g	2.5	Zinc	0.1mcg	0.7
Total fat	0.4g	0.5	Vitamin A	43.4mg	2.9
made up of:			Vitamin C	64.4mg	107.3
saturated	–	–	Vitamin D	–	–
polyunsat.	0.1g	–	Vitamin E	5.0mg	42.0
mono-unsat.	–	–	Vitamin B_1	0.3mg	33.8
Cholesterol	–	–	Vitamin B_2	0.1mg	7.5
Fibre	2.4g	8.0	Nicotinic Acid	0.7mg	4.5
Iron	2.8mg	26.8	Vitamin B_6	0.1mg	5.0
Calcium	49.6mg	10.0	Vitamin B_{12}	–	–
Magnesium	16.5mg	5.5	Folic Acid	35.3mg	11.8
Potassium	426.0mg	14.2	Starch	–	–
Sodium	28.2mg	2.3	Sugars	6.1g	–

USEFUL FOR: HYPERTENSION REDUCTION; COELIACS; DAIRY FOOD ALLERGY DIETS; CANCER PREVENTION; HEART DISEASE PREVENTION; STROKE PREVENTION.

TIP BOX

Cut the top off a tomato and carefully hollow out the middle. Stuff with a mixture of low fat soft cheese and herbs or with pulses and sprouted beans. Replace their 'caps' and serve with a salad.

101

Mange-Tout and Okra Salad (V 4)

A beautifully crisp and colourful salad which has a nice freshness about it.

Preparation Time: 15 minutes
Cooking Time: 5 minutes
Ingredients: Imperial/Metric
4oz/100g   okra, washed and topped
4oz/100g   carrot, washed
4oz/100g   mange-tout, washed and trimmed
2oz/50g   sunflower seeds
2oz/50g   spring onions, washed and curled

Method
1 Steam the okra for 5 minutes. Run under cold water to fix the colour.
2 Cut the carrots into long, thin sticks with a sharp knife.
3 Mix the first four ingredients together and place the 'curled' onions standing like weeping willows on the salad base. To curl the spring onions, wash them and trim off the roots and any discoloured or lanky outer leaves, so you have a nice straight green and white length. Then split the onion lengthways, almost to the base, making two downward cuts, one at right angles to the other, so the green part will curl downwards. Plunge into iced water for 15 minutes.

NUTRITION BOX (per serving)					
	Quantity	% RDA		Quantity	% RDA
Calories	65.3	2.6	Copper	0.1mcg	6.6
Protein	2.5g	4.0	Zinc	0.3mcg	2.5
Total fat	0.1g	0.2	Vitamin A	645.3mg	86.0
made up of:			Vitamin C	16.6mg	55.2
saturated	–	–	Vitamin D	–	–
polyunsat.	–	–	Vitamin E	4.0mg	33.6
mono-unsat.	–	–	Vitamin B$_1$	0.4mg	37.4
Cholesterol	–	–	Vitamin B$_2$	3.5mg	242.5
Fibre	4.0g	13.3	Nicotinic Acid	1.3mg	8.1
Iron	1.8mg	17.8	Vitamin B$_6$	0.1mg	4.8
Calcium	70.0mg	14.0	Vitamin B$_{12}$	–	–
Magnesium	33.3mg	11.1	Folic Acid	63.1mg	21.0
Potassium	272.2mg	9.1	Starch	1.9g	–
Sodium	19.4mg	1.6	Sugars	3.7g	–

USEFUL FOR: HYPERTENSION REDUCTION; COELIACS; HEART DISEASE PREVENTION; STROKE PREVENTION; CANCER PREVENTION; CHOLESTEROL REDUCTION; DAIRY FOOD ALLERGY DIETS.

9
FINISHING TOUCHES

To most people a meal without a sweet to end with is not a 'proper meal'. Personally, I like nothing better than fresh fruits of the season – either plain or in a fruit salad. But for many people used to traditional food, this is not enough.

My husband has a very sweet tooth and so over the years I have developed recipes for desserts which will satisfy him without being a health hazard. The traditional types of desserts are extremely unhealthy as they are usually very high in sugar and fats and low in fibre. The recipes in this chapter are all extremely low in fat and sugar and quite high in fibre. You will notice immediately that two of the most popular ingredients used for traditional sweets, cream and sugar, are absent from my recipes. Both are very easy to

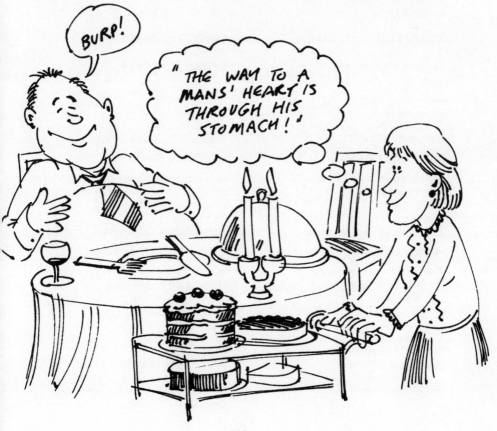

replace with healthier alternatives, but this does not mean that the desserts will be tart or lack flavour.

Take advantage of fresh seasonal fruits by using them in mousses and crumbles. There are many interesting and exotic fruits with which to experiment. I like to mix fresh fruits with dried fruits as this gives a nice texture to the dish and increases the fibre content. To serve with your dessert try low fat natural yogurt, tofu or a soya based topping instead of cream or custard.

Conversion Recipes

Converting traditional desserts into healthier versions is relatively easy. The main ingredients which usually have to be changed are sugar and cream.

The substitutes I use for sugar are dried dates, concentrated fruit juices and honey. These act as sweeteners but have fewer calories and more nutrients than sugar.

Instead of cream I use silken tofu, fromage frais, concentrated soya milk or low fat natural yogurt. The desserts will be just as rich and creamy as traditional ones made with cream but will have the benefit of fewer calories and far less fat.

These conversion recipes will give you an idea of the substitution process in action.

TRADITIONAL RECIPE

CONVERSION RECIPE

Country Plum Mould

1lb/500g plums
2tsp stem ginger
2tbsp sugar
3tsp gelatine
10fl oz/300ml cream

Country Plum Mould

1lb/500g plums
2tsp stem ginger
1tbsp honey
3tsp Gelozone
10fl oz/300ml fromage frais

Caledonian Cream

6tsp marmalade
2oz/30g sugar
4tbsp whisky
1 lemon, juice
10fl oz/300ml double cream

Caledonian Cream

6tsp marmalade (sugar-free)
1oz/15ml concentrated raspberry juice
4tbsp whisky or fruit juice
1 lemon juice
10fl oz/100ml silken tofu

Apple and Blackberry Tart

4oz/125g shortcrust pastry
1lb/500g cooking apples
2oz/50g butter

1 egg
2oz/50g sugar
1oz/25g sultanas
8oz/225g blackberries
½tsp cinnamon
6fl oz/150ml cream

Apple and Blackberry Tart

4oz/125g wholemeal, low fat pastry
1lb/500g cooking apples
2oz/50g polyunsaturated margarine,
unhydrogenated
1 egg white
2oz/50g dried dates
1oz/25g sultanas
8oz/225g blackberries
½tsp cinnamon
6fl oz/150ml low fat natural yogurt,
thick set

Dried Fruit Crumble (V 4)

Any combination of dried fruits can be used for this dish – experiment to find the flavour you like the best.

Preparation Time: 15 minutes
Cooking Time: 45 minutes
Temperature: 190°C, 375°F, Gas Mark 5
Ingredients: Imperial/Metric

4oz/125g	dried prunes
2oz/50g	currants
2oz/50g	raisins
2oz/50g	dried dates
1	fresh banana
1tsp	ground cinnamon
1tsp	mixed spice
10fl oz/250ml	unsweetened pineapple juice
8oz/200g	oats
2tbsp	honey

Method

1 Wash the dried fruit well.
2 Soak overnight in the fruit juice.
3 Place all the ingredients, except the oats and honey, in a saucepan and add the juice.
4 Bring to the boil and simmer for about 20 minutes – until the fruit is soft and the liquid has thickened.
5 Heat the honey and mix with the oats. Place the fruit in an ovenproof dish and pile on the topping. Cook in a preheated oven until brown and crispy – about 25 minutes.
6 Serve either hot or cold with natural unsweetened yogurt.

> **TIP BOX**
>
> Dates have been cultivated for over 5,000 years in the Middle East and are well known as a sugar substitute – both for wine and food. They are also a good source of nutrients and fibre.

NUTRITION BOX (per serving)					
	Quantity	% RDA		Quantity	% RDA
Calories	199.1	8.0	Copper	0.1mcg	6.6
Protein	2.6g	4.1	Zinc	0.5mcg	5.0
Total fat	1.4g	0.1	Vitamin A	16.5mg	2.2
made up of:			Vitamin C	2.5mg	8.3
saturated	0.2g	–	Vitamin D	–	–
polyunsat.	0.5g	–	Vitamin E	0.1mg	1.1
mono-unsat.	0.6g	–	Vitamin B_1	0.3mg	26.3
Cholesterol	–	–	Vitamin B_2	0.1mg	3.5
Fibre	3.6g	12.2	Nicotinic Acid	0.8mg	4.8
Iron	1.4mg	13.6	Vitamin B_6	0.1mg	4.7
Calcium	29.5mg	5.9	Vitamin B_{12}	–	–
Magnesium	31.6mg	10.5	Folic Acid	11.6mg	3.9
Potassium	317.2mg	10.5	Starch	11.4g	–
Sodium	11.7mg	1.0	Sugars	22.2g	–

USEFUL FOR: DAIRY FOOD ALLERGY DIETS; HYPERTENSION REDUCTION.

TIP BOX

Fruits with tough skins and pips contain more fibre than fleshy soft fruits.

Pineapple Cheesecake (F 4)
You can ring the changes with this recipe by making the base from bran and honey. It is also an excellent dessert for a formal dinner party.

Preparation Time: 45 minutes
Cooking Time: 35 minutes
Temperature: 170°C, 340°F, Gas Mark 3
Ingredients: Imperial/Metric
2oz/50g	polyunsaturated margarine (unhydrogenated)
8oz/225g	medium oats, toasted
3tbsp	honey
12oz/350g	low fat vegetarian soft cheese
½oz/15g	wholemeal flour
1	lemon, zest and juice
1oz/25g	sunflower seeds, ground
3	egg whites
1lb/500g	pineapple, peeled and chopped into segments

Method

1 Make the base by melting the margarine and mixing with the oats and 1 tbsp of the honey. Pack this mixture hard into the base of a loose sided flan or cake tin.
2 Beat the cheese until softened.
3 Add the flour, lemon juice, rind, remaining honey and ground seeds.
4 Beat the egg whites until stiff and carefully fold in to the mixture.
5 Spread this carefully over the oat base and level.
6 Arrange pineapple segments attractively on top of the mixture.
7 Bake in a preheated oven until heated through and just beginning to turn a very pale golden brown – about 35 minutes.
8 Cover with foil towards the end of the cooking period if it looks like being too brown.
9 Leave to cool completely on a wire tray before removing from the tin.

TIP BOX

Yellow melons, peaches and apricots are the best source of vitamin A in fruit.

NUTRITION BOX (per serving)					
	Quantity	% RDA		Quantity	% RDA
Calories	273.0	11.0	Copper	0.1mcg	5.8
Protein	9.1g	15.0	Zinc	1.0mcg	9.6
Total fat	11.5g	15.4	Vitamin A	62.5mg	8.3
made up of:			Vitamin C	18.8mg	62.5
saturated	1.7g	–	Vitamin D	0.5mcg	4.9
polyunsat.	2.7g	–	Vitamin E	2.8mg	23.1
mono-unsat.	2.3g	–	Vitamin B_1	0.3mg	26.1
Cholesterol	–	–	Vitamin B_2	0.1mg	3.5
Fibre	6.6g	22.0	Nicotinic Acid	1.0mg	6.2
Iron	1.7mg	17.0	Vitamin B_6	0.1mg	4.7
Calcium	27.9mg	5.5	Vitamin B_{12}	0.3mcg	15.6
Magnesium	45.5mg	15.1	Folic Acid	24.8mcg	8.3
Potassium	306.5mg	10.2	Starch	22.8g	–
Sodium	61.1mg	5.1	Sugars	16.9g	–
USEFUL FOR: HYPERTENSION REDUCTION; CANCER PREVENTION; STROKE PREVENTION; CHOLESTEROL REDUCTION; HEART DISEASE PREVENTION					

Plum Crunch (F V 8)

This was invented for my dad who loves plums in tarts and crumbles but has always eaten them made with lots of white sugar and white flour. This tastes better and is far healthier.

Preparation Time: 30 minutes
Cooking Time: 40 minutes
Temperature: 170°C, 340°F, Gas Mark 3
Ingredients: Imperial/Metric

1lb/450g	eating plums, washed, stoned and halved
4tbsp	honey
2oz/50g	polyunsaturated margarine (unhydrogenated)
4oz/100g	wholemeal flour
2oz/50g	barley flakes
1oz/25g	jumbo oats
2tbsp	sunflower seeds
2tbsp	sesame oil

Method

1 Place the plums in a large, shallow ovenproof dish.
2 Warm the honey and pour 2tbsp over the plums.
3 Rub the margarine into the flour until the mixture resembles fine breadcrumbs.
4 Add the barley flakes, jumbo oats and seeds.
5 Add the rest of the warm honey and stir into the mixture.
6 Add the oil and mix well.
7 Place on top of the plum mixture and cook in a preheated oven until the topping is golden brown and crisp, about 40 minutes.

NUTRITION BOX (per serving)					
	Quantity	% RDA		Quantity	% RDA
Calories	194.7	7.8	Copper	–	4.2
Protein	2.9g	4.7	Zinc	0.7mcg	6.6
Total fat	10.0g	13.4	Vitamin A	60.9mg	8.1
made up of:			Vitamin C	0.4mg	1.2
saturated	2.0g	–	Vitamin D	0.5mcg	4.9
polyunsat.	3.5g	–	Vitamin E	3.2mg	26.7
mono-unsat.	4.4g	–	Vitamin B_1	0.2mg	18.4
Cholesterol	–	–	Vitamin B_2	–	2.4
Fibre	2.0g	6.6	Nicotinic Acid	0.7mg	4.0
Iron	1.2mg	12.1	Vitamin B_6	0.1mg	3.9
Calcium	16.0mg	3.2	Vitamin B_{12}	0.3mcg	15.6
Magnesium	30.3mg	10.0	Folic Acid	30.0mg	10.0
Potassium	141.8mg	4.7	Starch	14.8g	–
Sodium	54.5mg	4.5	Sugars	51.9g	–
USEFUL FOR: DAIRY FOOD ALLERGY DIET.					

Prune and Banana Yogurt (4)
A lovely rich creamy dessert that is quick to make and very healthy!

Preparation Time: 10 minutes
Chilling Time: Overnight
Ingredients: Imperial/Metric
4oz/100g   prunes, washed and pitted
1   banana
10fl oz/250ml natural unsweetened low fat yogurt

Method
1 Chop the prunes
2 Slice the banana
3 Mix the yogurt with the prunes and banana
4 Pile the mixture into a serving dish and leave in the refrigerator overnight
   to thicken.
5 Serve chilled.

NUTRITION BOX (per serving)					
	Quantity	% RDA		Quantity	% RDA
Calories	77.9	3.1	Copper	0.1mcg	4.5
Protein	3.9g	6.3	Zinc	0.4mcg	4.3
Total fat	.7g	9.3	Vitamin A	40.4mg	5.4
made up of:			Vitamin C	2.8mg	9.2
saturated	–	–	Vitamin D	–	–
polyunsat.	–	–	Vitamin E	0.1mg	0.4
mono-unsat.	1.7g	–	Vitamin B$_1$	0.3mg	34.4
Cholesterol	4.3g	–	Vitamin B$_2$	0.4mg	25.2
Fibre	2.8g	9.3	Nicotinic Acid	0.9mg	5.6
Iron	0.6mg	5.8	Vitamin B$_6$	0.2mg	7.6
Calcium	120.9mg	24.0	Vitamin B$_{12}$	–	–
Magnesium	25.9mg	8.4	Folic Acid	6.8mg	2.2
Potassium	375.0mg	12.5	Starch	0.8g	–
Sodium	49.9mg	4.2	Sugars	10.5g	–
USEFUL FOR: HYPERTENSION REDUCTION; COELIACS.					

TIP BOX

Fresh fruits consist of between 80-90%
water.

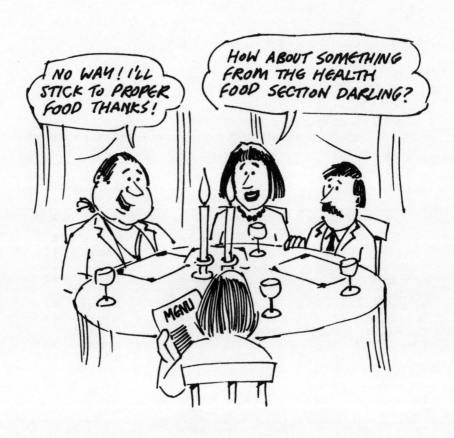

10
YOU CAN HAVE YOUR CAKE AND EAT IT!

You may be asking yourself how a chapter on cakes, of all things, finds its way into a book that is concerned solely with healthy eating. Cakes are seen as being a treat, naughty but nice, in which to indulge from time to time. And then, perhaps, you feel guilty afterwards, for surely all sugar, butter, white flour and eggs that form the basis of a cake, must be bad for the health? Well, yes, these ingredients are bad for our health in one way or another, but almost everything in a cake that is unhealthy can be replaced by something that is better for our health.

Eating a healthy diet definitely does not mean that you have to abstain from enjoying cakes. And I do mean ENJOY. Many people believe that a healthier type of cake, by its very nature, must be so heavy that it sinks to the base of your stomach like a lead balloon. It is regarded as something to be endured and certainly not enjoyed. Admittedly, Richard and I have encountered such cakes in many a health food restaurant and in my opinion they should sport a government health warning.

I enjoy a nice piece of cake with a cup of tea – and Richard certainly does – so over the years I have developed a whole range of cakes which are not only delicious but healthy as well. Most of them can also double up as puddings – especially if you warm the slices up in a microwave or gently steam them over a pan of boiling water for a few minutes. This transforms the cakes into light, fluffy desserts which taste wonderful with some concentrated soya milk poured over them.

Quite often I experiment by using vegetables as the base for a cake recipe. Would you believe that you can make a cake with grated courgettes? Such a cake was among the food which I had taken along to a Miriam Stoppard Show in which I was appearing and the film crew absolutely loved it. They could not believe that it was an example of a healthy cake – it tasted too good! So don't be deterred, you really can have your cake and eat it!

Common problems
Basically, there are two common problems which people seem to experience when making a 'healthy' cake: the cake is either too dry or too heavy.

I am often asked why a 'healthy' cake is extremely dry and, therefore, crumbly. There is nothing as discouraging as slicing a cake and watching each slice disintegrate into a pile of crumbs. Nor is it very impressive.

The cause is simple and extremely easy to remedy. If you use wholemeal flour instead of white you should add a little extra liquid to the mixture.

This is because wholemeal flours are much more dense and so absorb more liquid than their white counterparts. There is no strict rule as to how much extra liquid is needed as each type of flour will vary. Even different batches of the same flour will vary in absorbency. However, a good yardstick is to check the consistency of the mixture which should be firm enough to stick to a tablespoon and yet runny enough to drop off the spoon fairly easily. Remember that when you subsitute honey, or a dried date purée, for sugar you are also adding extra liquid. You will adapt very quickly to this new method of cake making until, before you know it, you do it without even thinking.

A cake that is too heavy can be quite unpalatable and, once again, it seems to be synonymous with a healthy cake. Again the main culprit is the wholemeal flour. The bran and husk of the grain are retained in wholemeal flour which makes it heavier than the white processed type. Cakes do, therefore, have a tendency to be heavier if made with wholemeal flour.

However, there are certain steps you can take to remedy this problem. Try mixing the wholemeal flour with other types, such as barley flour, brown rice flour or even white flour, as this will help 'lighten' the cake. Many people will no doubt complain if I advocate the use of white flour. I justify its use because people can become so discouraged with trying to eat a healthy diet that they abandon the attempt completely. This defeats the object and so I see little wrong in a compromise. The idea is to improve your diet. In my opinion it is far better to use 50% white flour than reverting to 100%.

You can also 'lighten' a cake by adding one or two teaspoons of low sodium baking powder to the flour or by using 85%, rather than 100%, wholemeal flour. The 100% variety is heavier because it contains all the bran, germ and husk of the wheat grain, whereas the other variety contains only 85%. It is surprising what a difference the use of this lighter flour makes to the cake.

Healthy eating should be enjoyable, not something to 'put up with' for the sake of your health, and cakes are no exception.

Conversion Recipes
No doubt you will have made cakes that have become firm favourites with your family and, understandably, you will feel a little reluctant to toss them to one side. Well, it is often quite easy to make that old familiar cake much more healthy by simply making one or two changes to the ingredients. And once you are familiar with the process, it will become second nature to you.

To give you an idea of exactly what I mean I have 'converted' three traditional cake recipes, which are probably familiar to you, into much healthier versions of the same thing. Using this technique you will be able to 'convert' any recipe you wish.

But, remember, there are no hard and fast rules about the conversion process and it does tend to boil down to trial and error in the end. However, my conversion guide should help to minimize the errors. The different methods and techniques which may be required are explained in the recipes later in the chapter.

TRADITIONAL RECIPE	CONVERSION RECIPE

Victoria Sandwich

Victoria Sandwich	Victoria Sandwich
6oz butter	6oz polyunsaturated margarine (unhydrogenated)
6oz caster sugar	3oz honey
3 eggs	3 egg whites
	1½tbsp tahini (sesame seed paste)
6oz self raising flour	5oz plain wholemeal flour
	1oz soya flour
	3tsp baking powder (low sodium)
3tbsp jam	3tbsp jam (sugar free)

Dark Ginger Cake	Dark Ginger Cake
6oz treacle	6oz dried dates, puréed
2oz sugar	2oz blackstrap molasses
3oz butter	3oz polyunsaturated margarine (unhydrogenated)
6oz flour	5oz plain wholemeal flour
	1oz soya flour
	2tsp baking powder (low sodium)
2tsp ground ginger	same
1tsp mixed spice	same
1tsp bicarbonate of soda	not required
3 eggs	3 egg whites
	1½tbsp tahini (sesame seed paste)
4tbsp milk	4tbsp skimmed, or soya milk
Butter frosting:	Healthy frosting:
3oz butter	½pt low fat natural unsweetened yogurt
6oz icing sugar	3oz dried prunes (soaked in yogurt overnight)

Chocolate Cream Gateau	Chocolate Cream Gateau
4 eggs	4 egg whites
	2tbsp tahini (sesame seed paste)
4oz caster sugar	2oz honey
3oz self-raising flour	3oz wholemeal flour
	1tsp baking powder (low sodium)
3oz butter	3oz polyunsaturated oil (cold pressed)
Filling and topping:	Filling and topping:
½pt double cream	¾pt silken tofu
¼pt single cream	not required
½tsp vanilla essence	½tsp natural vanilla essence
4oz caster sugar	3oz dried dates (soaked in tofu overnight)

Marrow and Orange Cake (F 8)

Everyone thought I had gone too far with this one – until they tasted it!

Preparation Time: 25 minutes
Cooking Time: 65 minutes
Temperature: 180°C, 350°F, Gas Mark 4
Ingredients: Imperial/Metric

6oz/175g	marrow, peeled, deseeded and cut into small cubes
4oz/100g	polyunsaturated margarine (unhydrogenated)
3oz/75g	honey
2	eggs whites
1	orange (very well scrubbed) zest and juice
10oz/275g	wholemeal flour
4tsp	baking powder (low sodium)
1	orange, peeled and sliced

Method

1 Oil and line a 20cm (8in) cake tin.
2 Steam marrow for 10 minutes. Leave to cool.
3 Beat together the margarine and honey until thoroughly mixed.
4 Add egg whites gradually, beating well.
5 Add orange rind, juice and marrow. Stir well.
6 Sift the flour and baking powder. Stir well.
7 Spoon the mixture into the prepared tin.
8 Arrange the orange slices on top of the cake.
9 Bake until well risen and golden brown, about 1 hour. Turn out and cool on a wire rack.

NUTRITION BOX (per serving)					
	Quantity	% RDA		Quantity	% RDA
Calories	243	9.8	Copper	0.21mcg	10.3
Protein	4.9g	7.9	Zinc	1.1mcg	10.6
Total fat	11.3g	15.3	Vitamin A	113.6mg	15.1
made up of:			Vitamin C	23.5mg	78.3
saturated	2.7g	–	Vitamin D	1.0mcg	9.9
polyunsat.	5.7g	–	Vitamin E	3.5mg	28.9
mono-unsat.	2.5g	–	Vitamin B_1	0.18mg	18.2
Cholesterol	–	–	Vitamin B_2	0.06mg	4.3
Fibre	4.7g	15.8	Nicotinic Acid	1.0mg	6.3
Iron	2.1mg	20.4	Vitamin B_6	0.2mg	6.3
Calcium	47.1mg	9.4	Vitamin B_{12}	0.63mcg	31.25
Magnesium	52.6mg	17.5	Folic Acid	30.1mg	10.0
Potassium	212.7mg	7.1	Starch	21.8g	–
Sodium	103.8mg	8.6	Sugars	132.7g	–
USEFUL FOR: CANCER PREVENTION; HEART DISEASE PREVENTION; STROKE PREVENTION; MILK ALLERGY DIETS; CHOLESTEROL REDUCTION.					

Pineapple Fruit Cake (F V 8)

An unusual combination of dried and fresh fruit that tastes refreshingly different. The cake is nice and moist and cuts well. It also keeps very well, provided you wrap it carefully in greaseproof paper and foil.

Preparation Time: 35 minutes
Cooking Time: 15 minutes
Temperature: 160°C, 325°F, Gas Mark 3
Ingredients: Imperial/Metric

6oz/175g	dried dates
4oz/100g	raisins
4oz/100g	currants
4oz/100g	pineapple, fresh if possible otherwise use tinned without added sugar, but drain well
4oz/100g	grated carrot
7oz/200g	wholemeal flour
3tsp	baking powder (low sodium)
2	lemons (very well scrubbed) zest
7tbsp	pineapple juice, unsweetened

Topping

2tbsp	pineapple juice, unsweetened
½tsp	Gelozone
1oz/25g	pineapple, chopped

Method

1 Grease a 20cm (8in) round cake tin.
2 Place the dates in a small saucepan with just enough boiling water to cover. Bring to the boil and simmer for about 10 minutes until soft and pulpy. Leave to cool slightly.
3 Mix together the dried fruit, pineapple, carrot, flour, baking powder and lemon zest.
4 Add the juice and date mixture.
5 Spoon into the prepared tin and bake in a preheated oven until firm to the touch – about 1 hour and 15 minutes.
6 To make the topping: gently heat the pineapple juice. Sprinkle on the Gelozone and whisk vigorously. Do not allow to boil. Once the juice begins to steam it will be ready. Add the pineapple chunks and spread the mixture over the fruit cake whilst it is still warm.

TIP BOX

I find that the quickest way to remove the zest from an orange is with a utensil called a 'zester'. It not only saves time and effort but looks more attractive as well.

NUTRITION BOX (per serving)					
	Quantity	% RDA		Quantity	% RDA
Calories	309	12.4	Copper	0.27mcg	13.3
Protein	4.3g	6.8	Zinc	0.87mcg	8.9
Total fat	0.5g	0.7	Vitamin A	255.2mg	7.1
made up of:			Vitamin C	5.9mg	19.8
saturated	0.07g	–	Vitamin D	–	–
polyunsat.	0.22g	–	Vitamin E	0.31mg	2.6
mono-unsat.	–	–	Vitamin B_1	0.17mg	17.0
Cholesterol	–	–	Vitamin B_2	0.06mg	4.1
Fibre	6.4g	21.2	Nicotinic Acid	1.5mg	9.4
Iron	1.9mg	19.0	Vitamin B_6	0.14mg	7.1
Calcium	50.8mg	10.2	Vitamin B_{12}	–	–
Magnesium	62.2mg	20.7	Folic Acid	23.4mg	7.8
Potassium	513.4mg	17.1	Starch	15.9g	–
Sodium	17.5mg	1.4	Sugars	123.5g	–

USEFUL FOR: CANCER PREVENTION; HEART DISEASE
PREVENTION; DAIRY FOOD ALLERGY DIETS; CHOLESTEROL
REDUCTION; HYPERTENSION REDUCTION.

Sticky Prune and Date Cake (F 8)

If, like me, you enjoy sticky, substantial cakes then you will love this recipe.
It is particularly good served with natural low fat yogurt. The prunes give
the cake a natural laxative effect because they contain a natural substance
similar to biscodyl – the active ingredient in many laxatives and
suppositories!

Preparation Time: 35 minutes
Cooking Time: 45 minutes
Temperature: 180°C, 350°F, Gas Mark 4
Ingredients: Imperial/Metric
4oz/125g   dried dates, washed and pitted
4oz/125g   dried prunes, washed and pitted
4fl oz/125ml sesame seed oil (cold pressed)
1   egg white
1tbsp   tahini
5oz/150g   wholemeal flour
2tsp   baking powder (low sodium)
½tsp   freshly grated nutmeg
1tsp   ground cinnamon
3fl oz/75ml soya milk

Topping:
2tbsp   soya milk
1tbsp   honey
1tbsp   blackstrap molasses
             few drops natural vanilla essence

116

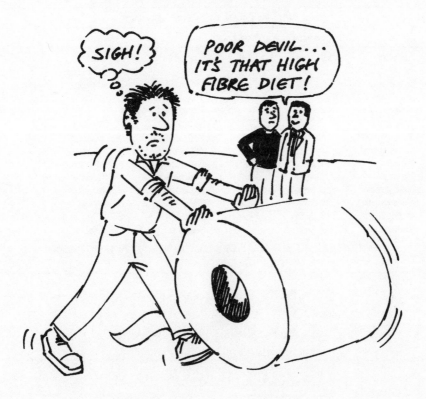

Method

1 Oil and line a 20cm (8in) round cake tin.
2 Place dates in a saucepan and just cover with water. Bring to the boil and simmer until the dates are soft and pulpy. Do the same in another saucepan with the prunes. Leave both to cool slightly.
3 Drain the prunes and chop roughly.
4 In a bowl whisk together dates, oil, egg whites and tahini until the mixture is thick and fluffy.
5 Sift the flour, baking powder and spices. Stir into the date mixture.
6 Add prunes and milk.
7 Pour mixture into the tin and bake in a preheated oven for 45 minutes until firm to the touch.
8 Warm all the topping ingredients together in a pan.
9 Once the cake is removed from the oven prick the top all over with a skewer and pour the warm topping over it.
10 Leave to cool in the tin. This is also nice served as a hot pudding with soya concentrated milk.

NUTRITION BOX (per serving)					
	Quantity	% RDA		Quantity	% RDA
Calories	296	11.8	Copper	0.12mcg	6.1
Protein	3.5g	5.6	Zinc	0.61mcg	6.1
Total fat	16.1g	21.5	Vitamin A	14.5mg	10.7
made up of:			Vitamin C	0.15mg	.5
saturated	2.2g	–	Vitamin D	–	–
polyunsat.	2.0g	–	Vitamin E	0.98mg	8.2
mono-unsat.	11.7g	–	Vitamin B_1	0.32mg	32.2
Cholesterol	–	–	Vitamin B_3	0.12mg	8.2
Fibre	4.3g	14.3	Nicotinic Acid	1.0mg	6.1
Iron	1.6mg	15.2	Vitamin B_6	0.22mg	10.7
Calcium	50.6mg	10.2	Vitamin B_{12}	0.03mcg	1.4
Magnesium	38.5mg	12.8	Folic Acid	14.4mg	4.8
Potassium	343.2mg	11.4	Starch	11.9g	–
Sodium	7.8mg	0.65	Sugars	84.4g	–
USEFUL FOR: MILK ALLERGY DIETS; HYPERTENSION REDUCTION.					

TIP BOX

A cake cooked in a microwave looks completely different to one cooked conventionally. The texture is softer and is more reminiscent of a steamed pudding than a cake. But, remember, be careful not to overcook in the microwave or you could wind up with a cinder. I speak from experience! As soon as the cake begins to shrink away from the sides of the mould it should be ready.

11
ANYONE FOR AFTERNOON TEA?

The English tradition of afternoon tea has declined over the years as the pace of life quickens. But it is still nice (and good for you!) once in a while to relax for a few precious minutes with a cup of tea and a home-made treat.

The scones are particularly adaptable: try adding different dried fruits and fruit zests. And don't stop at sweet variations, try herbs and spices as well – herb scones are nice served with soups and salads.

Common problems

Why do wholemeal scones always crumble? Well, the answer is they don't have to. The problem arises because of the nature of wholemeal flour. White flour is much lighter than wholemeal because it has had all the bran and husk removed and, therefore, is less absorbent. The secret of non-crumbly scones is to add more liquid to the mixture when using wholemeal flour.

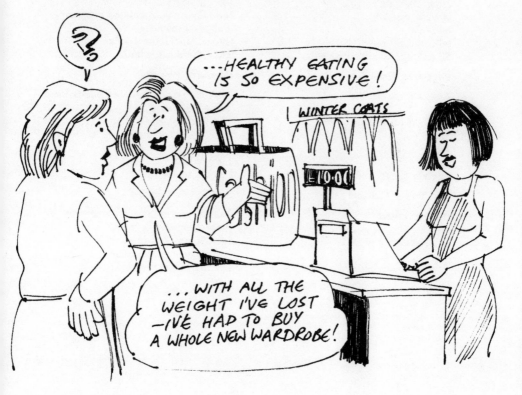

The dough should be firm, soft, pliable and should not crumble when you are rolling it out. When using a purée of dried dates to sweeten the scones you will automatically be using more liquid, so you must take this into account.

I like my scones to be heavy and substantial, but Richard doesn't. A reasonable compromise is to use three quarters wholemeal flour and a quarter white flour – you could even use half and half, or, as suggested in Chapter 10, use 85% wholemeal flour.

Conversion recipes

Converting scone and biscuit recipes is quite straightforward and most only require minimal changes. The main changes will tend to be concerned with dairy products and the type of flour used. The three recipes below will give you a good idea of what I mean.

TRADITIONAL RECIPE	CONVERSION RECIPE
Fruit Scones	**Fruit Scones**
12oz/350g self-raising flour	8oz/225g 85% wholemeal flour
	4oz/125g plain white flour
1tsp/5g salt	1tsp/5g low sodium salt
2tsp/10g baking powder	2tsp/10g low sodium baking powder
2tbsp/30g caster sugar	1oz/15g dried dates
3oz/75g butter	3oz /75g polyunsaturated margarine (unhydrogenated)
6fl oz/175ml milk	6fl oz/175l skimmed milk
5fl oz/150ml double cream	5floz/150ml silken tofu
Digestive Biscuits	**Digestive Biscuits**
4oz/100g butter	4oz/100g polyunsaturated margarine (unhydrogenated)
1lb/500g plain flour	1lb/500g wholemeal flour
1tsp/5g salt	1tsp/5g low sodium salt
1tbsp/5ml milk	
1 egg	1 egg white
2oz/50g sugar	1oz/25g honey
Nut Butter Cookies	**Nut Butter Cookies**
2oz/50g butter	2oz/50g polyunsaturated margarine (unhydrogenated)
2oz/50g caster sugar	1oz/25g raw brown sugar
3oz/75g flour	3oz/75g wholemeal flour
2oz/25g mixed nuts	2oz/50g mixed seeds

Apple Scone Ring (F V 8)

This is lovely toasted and eaten warm. I prefer the chopped apples to be quite 'chunky' as this gives a nice texture and you retain the distinctive flavours of the scone. You can, if you prefer, grate the apples and this will give a smoother scone with an even flavour throughout.

Preparation Time: 15 minutes
Cooking Time: 25 minutes
Temperature: 200°C, 400°F, Gas Mark 6
Ingredients: Imperial/Metric

1	cooking apple, large
8oz/225g	wholemeal flour
3tsp/3tsp	baking powder (low sodium)
2oz/50g	polyunsaturated margarine (unhydrogenated)
1oz/25g	honey
3fl oz/75ml	soya milk (sugar free)

Method

1 Peel, core and finely chop the apple.
2 Sift together the flour and baking powder.
3 Rub in the margarine.
4 Add the honey and chopped apple.
5 Add enough milk to form a soft dough.
6 On a lightly floured surface form into a large round 12mm (½in) thick and place on a greased baking tray.
7 Brush the top with a little milk and sprinkle with the raw brown sugar.
8 Bake in a preheated oven until risen and golden brown, about 25 minutes.

NUTRITION BOX (per serving)					
	Quantity	% RDA		Quantity	% RDA
Calories	159.3	6.3	Copper	0.1mcg	6.9
Protein	4.1g	6.6	Zinc	0.9mcg	8.7
Total fat	6.0g	8.0	Vitamin A	57.7mg	7.7
made up of:			Vitamin C	4.2mg	14.1
saturated	1.4g	–	Vitamin D	0.5mcg	4.9
polyunsat.	3.1g	–	Vitamin E	1.8mg	15.4
mono-unsat.	1.3g	–	Vitamin B$_1$	0.1mg	14.4
Cholesterol	–	–	Vitamin B$_2$	0.03mg	2.2
Fibre	3.2g	10.8	Nicotinic Acid	0.7mg	4.5
Iron	1.3mg	12.9	Vitamin B$_6$	0.2mg	10.3
Calcium	18.3mg	3.7	Vitamin B$_{12}$	0.3mcg	15.6
Magnesium	42.1mg	14.0	Folic Acid	17.4mg	5.8
Potassium	139.1mg	4.6	Starch	17.9g	–
Sodium	52.2mg	4.3	Sugars	106.3g	–
USEFUL FOR: DAIRY FOOD ALLERGY DIETS.					

Crunch Bites (F V 8)

Biscuits which are home-made bear no resemblance at all to shop bought versions. I like my biscuits to be crunchy and substantial – this recipe fits the bill very nicely.

Preparation Time: 20 minutes
Cooking Time: 15 minutes
Temperature: 180°C, 350°F, Gas Mark 4
Ingredients: Imperial/Metric

2oz/50g	dried dates, washed and pitted
4oz/100g	polyunsaturated margarine (unhydrogenated)
2oz/50g	honey
6oz/175g	wholemeal flour, self-raising
1oz/25g	jumbo oats
1oz/25g	barley flakes
1oz/25g	prunes, chopped
2oz/50g	sunflower seeds
1tsp	mixed spice, ground
1	orange, zest (well scrubbed)
1	lemon, zest (well scrubbed)
2tsp	baking powder (low sodium)

Method

1 Place the dates in a small saucepan with enough boiling water just to cover them. Simmer for 15 minutes until the dates are soft and pulpy. Leave to cool.
2 Melt the margarine.
3 Remove from the heat and stir in all the remaining ingredients.
4 Press the mixture into 8 evenly sized balls.
5 Place well apart on a greased baking sheet and flatten slightly.
6 Bake in a preheated oven for about 15 minutes until risen and golden brown.
7 Cool on a wire tray.

> ### TIP BOX
>
> If you are short of time and fancy home-baked biscuits, mix a little honey into some muesli, put teaspoonsful of this mixture on a lightly greased baking sheet and bake at 180°C/350°F/Gas Mark 4.

TIP BOX

Always use plain flour and add your
own low sodium baking powder. This
way you minimize the offending
sodium.

NUTRITION BOX (per serving)					
	Quantity	% RDA		Quantity	% RDA
Calories	232.5	9.3	Copper	0.2mcg	8.2
Protein	5.6g	9.0	Zinc	1.2mcg	12.3
Total fat	6.9g	9.2	Vitamin A	70.0mg	9.3
made up of:			Vitamin C	–	–
saturated	1.6g	–	Vitamin D	0.5mcg	5.0
polyunsat.	3.4g	–	Vitamin E	2.9mg	24.4
mono-unsat.	1.7g	–	Vitamin B_1	0.4mg	41.3
Cholesterol	–	–	Vitamin B_2	0.1mg	4.1
Fibre	5.1g	17.1	Nicotinic Acid	1.2mg	7.5
Iron	2.2mg	21.4	Vitamin B_6	0.2mg	8.1
Calcium	28.1mg	5.6	Vitamin B_{12}	0.3mcg	15.6
Magnesium	60.1mg	20.0	Folic Acid	24.8mg	8.3
Potassium	298.5mg	9.9	Starch	27.0g	–
Sodium	56.7mg	4.7	Sugars	110.8g	–

USEFUL FOR: DAIRY FOOD ALLERGY DIETS; HYPERTENSION
REDUCTION.

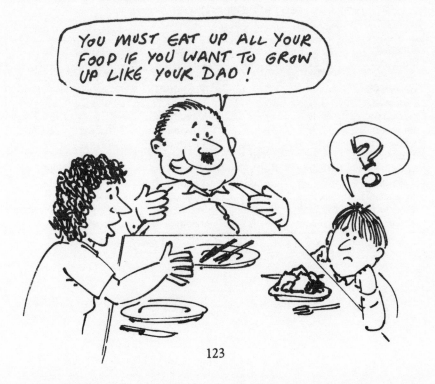

123

Fruit Scones (F V 8)

Try lemon and grapefruit as a change from the orange flavouring.

Preparation Time: 15 minutes
Cooking Time: 15 minutes
Temperature: 220°C, 420°F, Gas Mark 7
Ingredients: Imperial/Metric
8oz/225g   wholemeal flour
2tsp   baking powder (low sodium)
3oz/75g   polyunsaturated margarine (unhydrogenated)
1   orange, zest (well scrubbed) and juice
3oz/75g   raisins
½oz/12g   molasses
4fl oz/125ml soya milk

Method

1 Sieve the flour and baking powder into a bowl and rub in the margarine until the mixture resembles fine breadcrumbs.
2 Stir in the orange zest, juice, raisins, molasses and enough milk to make a fairly soft dough.
3 Knead the mixture gently on a lightly floured surface.
4 Roll out to a thickness of 25mm (1in) and cut into rounds with a cutter.
5 Place on a greased baking sheet and bake in a preheated oven for 15–20 minutes, until well risen and golden brown. Cool on a wire tray.

NUTRITION BOX (per serving)					
	Quantity	% RDA		Quantity	% RDA
Calories	266.1	10.6	Copper	0.1mcg	6.7
Protein	4.1g	6.6	Zinc	0.9mcg	8.6
Total fat	8.6g	11.5	Vitamin A	84.8mg	11.3
made up of:			Vitamin C	–	–
saturated	2.1g	–	Vitamin D	0.7mcg	7.4
polyunsat.	4.4g	–	Vitamin E	21.8mg	21.9
mono-unsat.	1.9g	–	Vitamin B_1	0.2mg	18.9
Cholesterol	–	–	Vitamin B_2	0.1mg	5.4
Fibre	3.1g	10.5	Nicotinic Acid	0.8mg	4.6
Iron	1.6mg	15.6	Vitamin B_6	0.3mg	13.8
Calcium	33.7mg	6.7	Vitamin B_{12}	0.5mcg	23.4
Magnesium	45.1mg	15.3	Folic Acid	16.4mg	5.5
Potassium	239.2mg	8.0	Starch	17.9g	–
Sodium	81.2mg	6.8	Sugars	108.3g	–
USEFUL FOR: DAIRY FOOD ALLERGY DIETS.					

Hot Poppy Seed Rolls (F V 8)

This must be my most 'asked for' recipe. These little round balls are full of flavour and look very attractive. They have a 'nutty', crunchy texture and are nice fresh from the oven, with a little 'healthy' margarine and low fat soft cheese.

Preparation Time: 10 minutes
Cooking Time: 20 minutes
Temperature: 230°C, 450°F, Gas Mark 8
Ingredients: Imperial/Metric
8oz/225g wholemeal flour
3tsp baking powder (low sodium)
¼tsp low sodium salt
2oz/50g polyunsaturated margarine (unhydrogenated)
2tbsp sunflower seeds, roasted
1tbsp poppy seeds
6tbsp soya milk

Method
1 Sift the flour, baking powder and salt into a bowl and rub in the margarine.
2 Add the seeds and mix well.
3 Mix in enough milk to give a soft dough.
4 Form into 8 evenly sized balls and place on a greased baking sheet.
5 Brush the tops with soya milk.
6 Bake in a preheated oven until well risen and golden brown, about 20 minutes.
7 Serve hot with soup or pâté.

NUTRITION BOX (per serving)					
	Quantity	% RDA		Quantity	% RDA
Calories	155.5	6.2	Copper	0.1mcg	5.6
Protein	4.1g	6.6	Zinc	0.8mcg	8.5
Total fat	6.0g	8.1	Vitamin A	56.3mg	7.5
made up of:			Vitamin C	–	–
saturated	1.4g	–	Vitamin D	0.5mcg	4.9
polyunsat.	3.1g	–	Vitamin E	3.6mg	29.9
mono-unsat.	1.5g	–	Vitamin B_1	0.2mg	24.4
Cholesterol	–	–	Vitamin B_2	0.04mg	2.6
Fibre	2.5g	8.3	Nicotinic Acid	0.7mg	4.3
Iron	1.6mg	16.0	Vitamin B_6	0.2mg	10.4
Calcium	25.1mg	5.0	Vitamin B_{12}	0.3mcg	15.6
Magnesium	43.7mg	14.6	Folic Acid	16.0mg	5.3
Potassium	156.0mg	5.2	Starch	17.8g	–
Sodium	51.4mg	4.3	Sugars	101.3g	–
USEFUL FOR: DAIRY FOOD ALLERGY DIETS.					

INDEX

apples: apple and blackberry tart, 104
  apple scone ring, 121
  melon, cheese and ginger refresher, 56
  spinach with apple, 95
  stuffed apples, 98
apricots, 107
arteries, blocked, 14, 16, 34–5
atherosclerosis, 34–5
aubergines: aubergine with tomatoes, 87–8
  chick pea moussaka, 68–9
  spiced vegetable bake, 79–80
  stuffed, 63–5

baking powder 123
banana and prune yogurt, 109
barley: cream of barley soup, 44
biscuits: crunch bites, 122–3
  digestive biscuits, 120
  nut butter cookies, 120
blackberry and apple tart, 104
blood, cholesterol levels, 16–17
blood pressure, 35–6
bread, 19, 20
breast cancer, 12
broccoli: broccoli with mint and yogurt, 88–9
  broccoli and mushroom pancake filling, 83
buckwheat flour, 81
  buckwheat pancake mixture, 82
butter beans: butter bean rissoles, 84
  leek and butter bean soup, 45

cabbage: stuffed Savoy, 74–5
cakes, 111–18
  chocolate cream gateau, 113
  dark ginger cake, 113
  marrow and orange cake, 114
  pineapple fruit cake, 115–16
  sticky prune and date cake, 116–18
  Victoria sandwich, 113
calcium, 30, 32, 35, 36
Caledonian cream, 104
calories, RDAs, 31
cancer, 11
  and fat consumption, 12–13
  and fibre, 20
  prevention, 36
caraway dumplings, 70–1

carrots: carrot and mushroom roulade, 66–7
  carrots with orange and ginger, 89–90
  tomato and carrot flan, 76–7
casserole with dumplings, 60–1
celery and cheese baked potato, 90–1
cheese soft: cheese and celery baked potato, 90–1
  herb dip, 49–50
  melon, cheese and ginger refresher, 56
  stuffed apples, 98
  vegetable lasagne, 77–8
cheesecake, pineapple, 106–7
chick peas: chick pea moussaka, 68–9
  hummus, 50–1
  spiced parcels, 62–3
chocolate cream gateau, 113
cholesterol, 13–14, 16–17, 20, 34–5
cobalamin, 28
Committee on Medical Aspects of Food Policy (COMA), 18–19
constipation, 19–20
conversion tables, 39–41
copper, 33
coronary artery disease, 34
country plum mould, 104
courgettes: courgette and melon salad, 99
courgettes with caraway dumplings, 70–1
  crunchy salad, 101
  vegetable pâté, 53–4
cranberries: festive loaf, 71–3
cream of barley soup, 44
creamy vegetable salad, 100
crumbles: dried fruit crumble, 105–6
  plum crunch, 108
  vegetable crumble, 80–1
crunch bites, 122–3
crunchy salad, 101

dairy products, 12, 18
dark ginger cake, 113
dates, 105
  crunch bites, 122–3
  sticky prune and date cake, 116–18
deficiency diseases, 11, 24
desserts, 103–9
digestive biscuits, 120
dips: garlic and tofu dip, 48
  herb dip, 49–50
  hummus, 50–51
Doll, Richard, 12

dried fruit: dried fruit crumble, 105–6
  pineapple fruit cake, 115–16
dumplings, 60–1
  caraway, 70–1

eczema, 12
Eskimos, 16
essential fatty acids, 16–17

fats, 15–18
  and cancer, 12–13, 16, 36
  and heart disease, 13–14, 16
  low fat spreads, 17–18
  mono-unsaturated, 17
  polyunsaturated, 16–18, 35
  saturated, 16, 18
festive loaf, 71–3
fibre, 18–20, 75
fish, 16, 18
flan, tomato and carrot, 76–7
folic acid, 29
French onion tart, 61
fromage frais: creamy vegetable salad, 100
  spiced vegetable bake, 79–80
fruit, vitamin content, 25–6
  see also dried fruit
fruit scones, 120, 124

garlic, 74, 80
  garlic and tofu dip, 48
  hummus, 50–1
ginger: carrots with orange and ginger, 89–90
  dark ginger cake, 113
  melon, cheese and ginger refresher, 56

heart attacks, 35
heart disease, 11, 13–14
  prevention, 34–5
herb dip, 49–50
high blood pressure, 14, 23, 35–6
hummus, 50–1

immune system, 36
iron, 30, 31, 32

lasagne, 60
  vegetable lasagne, 77–8
laxatives, 19
leeks: leek and butter bean soup, 45
  leeks with lemon and raisins, 92
legumes, 69
lemon: leeks with lemon and raisins, 92
  parsnip and lemon soup, 47–8
lentil pâté, 51–2
lettuce soup, 46
low fat pastry, 61–2
low fat spreads, 17–18

magnesium, 32, 35, 36
mange-tout: mange-tout and mushrooms, 93

mange-tout and okra salad, 102
margarine, 17
marrow and orange cake, 114
meat, 12, 18, 37
melon, 42–3, 107
  courgette and melon salad, 99
  melon, cheese and ginger refresher, 56
microwave ovens, 118
minerals, 30–3, 34
mint: broccoli with mint and yogurt, 88–9
mono-unsaturated fats, 16, 17
moussaka, chick pea, 68–9
mushrooms: broccoli and mushrooms
    pancake filling, 83
  carrot and mushroom roulade, 66–7
  chick pea moussaka, 68–9
  chopped mushroom pâté, 43
  festive loaf, 71–3
  mange-tout and mushrooms, 93
  mushroom and seed pâté, 52–3
  mushroom stroganoff, 73–4
  okra and mushrooms, 94
  stuffed Savoy, 74–5

nasturtium, 54
National Advisory Committee on Nutritional
    Education (NACNE), 15–16, 19, 21,
    23
nicotinic acid (niacin), 27, 35
nut butter cookies, 120
nutrition boxes, 38–9

oats: pineapple cheesecake, 106–7
oily fish, 16
okra: mange-tout and okra salad, 102
  okra and mushrooms, 94
olive oil, 17
onion tart, French, 61
orange: carrots with orange and ginger,
    89–90
  marrow and orange cake, 114
  zest, 115
oven temperatures, 40

pancakes: broccoli and mushroom pancake
    filling 83
  buckwheat pancake mixture, 82
pantothenic acid, 28
parsnip and lemon soup, 47–8
pastry, low fat, 61–2
pâtés, 42, 43
  chopped mushroom pâté, 43
  mushroom and seed pâté, 52–3
  soft lentil pâté, 51–2
  vegetable pâté, 53–4
peaches, 107
peas, split see split peas
peppers: vegetable crumble, 80–1
  vegetable lasagne, 77–8
phosphorus, 33